BONE MARROW TRANSPLANTATION IN EUROPE

BONE MARROW TRANSPLANTATION IN EUROPE

Proceedings of the Second European Symposium
on Bone Marrow Transplantation,
Courchevel, Savoie, France, March 27-30, 1978

Editor
Jean-Louis Touraine
Claude Bernard University, Lyon

Assistant Editors

R. Triau
General Secretary,
Fondation Mérieux, Lyon

F.E. Zwaan
General Secretary,
EBMT Group, Leiden

This publication was made possible by a grant
from the Fondation Mérieux

 1979

EXCERPTA MEDICA Amsterdam-Oxford-Princeton

ISBN Excerpta Medica 90 219 0399 7
ISBN Elsevier North-Holland 0 444 90113 2

Library of Congress Cataloging in Publication Data

European Symposium on Bone Marrow Transplantation,
2d, Courchevel, France, 1978.
Bone marrow transplantation in Europe.
Includes bibliographies and index.
1.   Marrow--Transplantation--Congresses.
I.   Touraine, Jean Louis.   II.   Triau, R.
III.   Zwaan, F. E.   IV.   Title.
RD123.5.E92   1978   617'.44   79-23852
ISBN 0-444-90113-2

Publisher:
Excerpta Medica
305 Keizersgracht
1000 BC Amsterdam
P.O. Box 1126

Sole Distributors for the USA and Canada:
Elsevier North-Holland Inc.
52 Vanderbilt Avenue
New York, N.Y. 10017

Printed in The Netherlands by Groen, IJmuiden

Preface

Two decades ago, the pioneering efforts of several investigators (1—3) established the feasibility of bone marrow transplantation in man and its potential as a treatment for irradiation accidents, aplastic anaemias, immunodeficiencies and acute leukaemias. Significant progress in our knowledge of histocompatibility and transplantation immunobiology and in clinical experience were necessary before bone marrow transplantation could be regarded as a therapeutic measure of relatively wide use and value. In the present era of marrow transplant expansion, as in the past, collaboration between haematologists, immunologists, paediatricians, pathologists, microbiologists, etc. from all countries is of the utmost importance. The goal of the First (4) and the Second European Symposia on Bone Marrow Transplantation, held in Courchevel, was to bring together physicians and scientists from several neighbouring countries, thus giving them the opportunity to share their experience in human marrow transplantation.

Although marrow transplantation is being increasingly used (an estimated 1000 patients have already been treated with marrow transplantation worldwide), the experience of each group is still limited. Informal exchange of precise information, especially between specialists working in different fields, was felt to be useful, interesting and necessary. This informal meeting was not intended to compete in any way with the International Marrow Transplantation meetings with their larger audience but rather to set the stage for practical collaboration between easily connected clinics or laboratories.

Methods for marrow transplantation in immunodeficiencies, aplastic anaemias and acute leukaemias are somewhat different as far as the conditioning regimen, the subsequent treatment and laboratory monitoring are concerned. Rejection of a marrow transplant does not occur in severe combined immunodeficiencies. Incomplete immune reconstitution is a problem in haematology but more so in primary immunodeficiencies. However, most immunobiological aspects (histocompatibility, prevention and treatment of graft-versus-host disease), isolation measures, and anti-infection therapies are common preoccupations and justify common efforts.

The overall European experience, as worldwide results contained in the International Bone Marrow Transplant Registry (5), shows the best results in severe combined immunodeficiency diseases: 56% long-lasting success with apparently definitive reconstitution. In the absence of a compatible donor, fetal tissue transplantation has resulted in immunological reconstitution of several patients, but the data are still too scarce and recent to allow a general analysis. In aplastic anaemia, marrow transplantation has proved successful in 36% of cases (with more than one year follow-up) and encouraging results have been obtained with antilymphocyte globulin treatment whether given alone or in conjunction with marrow infusion. All results reported reflect some progress in preceding years (4) and the latest data show even better improvement. In acute leukaemia, allogeneic marrow transplantation has not yet provided comparable results but hopes are being raised by modifications in irradiation and chemotherapy. Infusion of autologous marrow, possibly treated in vitro, may prove to be an interesting alternative. More details on these various forms of therapies will be found in the following reports.

It is the hope of all participants that the fruitful exchange of ideas on human marrow transplantation will continue to be very active and stimulating. It is their wish to gratefully acknowledge the help of the Fondation Mérieux. It is their goal to pursue the patient and international efforts which will make marrow transplantation a regularly successful form of treatment and leukaemia a curable disease. 'It is medicine's oldest dilemma, not to be settled by candor or by any kind of rhetoric; what it needs is a lot of time and patience, waiting for science to come in, as it has in the past, with the solid facts' (6).

Jean-Louis Touraine

References

1. Mathe, G., Schwarzenberg, L., Amiel, J.L. et al. (1959): Transfusions et greffes de moelle osseuse homologue chez des humains irradiés à haute dose accidentellement. *Rev. franç. Etud. clin. biol., 4,* 226.
2. Van Bekkum, D.W. and De Vries, M.J. (1967): *Radiation Chimaeras.* Academic Press, New York.
3. Thomas, E.D., Storb, R., Clift R.A. et al. (1975): Bone marrow transplantation. *New. Engl. J. Med., 292,* 832.
4. Bone Marrow Transplantation: Clinical Aspects (1978): Meeting of the Immunodeficiency Group and European Bone Marrow Transplantation Group, organized by E. Gluckman and J.L. Touraine. *Path. et Biol., 26,* 13.
5. Bortin, M.M. and Rimm, A.A. (1977): Severe combined immunodeficiency disease: Characterization of the disease and results of transplantation. *Transplantat. Proc., 9,* 169.
6. Thomas, L. (1978): Notes of a biology-watcher. On magic in medicine. *New. Engl. J. Med., 299,* 461.

Contents

I. Aplastic anaemia

THE PATTERN OF HEMOPOIETIC RECONSTITUTION AFTER ALG AND
BONE MARROW INFUSION IN SEVERE APLASTIC ANEMIA[x]

P. Cornu, B. Speck, W. Weber, C. Nissen, J. Sartorius[o] and
P. Groff

Division of Hematology, Department of Internal Medicine,
Kantonsspital Basel and Kinderspital Basel[o], Switzerland

SUMMARY

Immunosuppression with ALG (anti-lymphocyte-globulin) with or without
marrow infusion from a haploidentical family donor has become a real
alternative in the treatment of severe aplastic anemia for patients
without histocompatible sibling.
    Nine of 13 patients of the reported series are long-term survivors
with almost complete autologous reconstitutions. All these patients
experienced reconstitution 1-4 months after conditioning and restarting
of the androgens. All the patients who died had not been restarted on
androgens after immunosuppression and bone marrow infusion. Time factor
and androgens appear to be essential in autologous reconstitutions following immunosuppression with ALG followed by marrow infusion.

Immunosuppression with anti-lymphocyte-globulin (ALG) followed or not by bone marrow infusion in severe aplastic
anemia (SAA) has now become a real alternative to bone
marrow transplantation (BMT) in patients without histocompatible sibling. Survival with sustained remission has been
observed in over 50% of the cases as described recently
(1,2).
    Whether marrow infusion improves the results or not is
still not clear. The answer should come from the randomized
trial of the European Cooperative Group for BMT (EBMT) which
is currently underway.
    We would like to summarize here our experience with
ALG and marrow infusion and try to emphasize some special
aspects of autologous reconstitution.

MATERIAL AND METHODS

1. Patients

We have now treated 14 patients, who all fulfilled the criteria of SAA. All received ALG and marrow infusion as described later, 1 patient is too early for evaluation. The
median age of the patient was 14.0 years with a range of
4-50 years. Median duration of the disease prior to ALG and

[x]Supported by the Swiss Cancer League Grants FOR 080.AK.75 and FOR
   101.AK.77 (2) and the Swiss Science Foundation Grant 3.3320.74.

3

marrow was 6 months with a range of 2-38 months.

All the patients were on androgens, oxymetholone in most cases, prior to ALG. Two patients had an initial response, one of them under a very high dose of etiocholanolone. Both became refractory after 1½ year of treatment. The median duration of androgen therapy prior to immunosuppression with ALG was 3 months with a range of 1-30 months. Most of the patients received more than 20 transfusions from different donors. All patients with more than 20 transfusions were refractory to random platelets. One patient was not transfused at all. She maintained a hemoglobin of 4 g% for 1 year before a rapid deterioration began and all criteria of SAA were fulfilled.

2. Immunosuppression and marrow infusion

All the patients received 4 x 40 mg/kg body weight ALG (Lymphoser Berna, Schweiz. Serum- und Impfinstitut Bern) on consecutive days as an i.v. infusion over 3 hours under prophylactic platelet transfusion from unrelated best compatible donors. Marrow from a haploidentical family donor was infused 48 hours after the last ALG. Mean marrow cells number was 2.8 x 10^8/kg body weight (range: 1.8-4.9 x 10^8).

Supportive care was provided as for patients undergoing BMT after cyclophosphamide conditioning: platelets were transfused prophylactically by values under 20,000/mm^3, red cells were transfused in order to maintain hemoglobin levels between 8 and 10 g%. Granulocyte transfusions were performed in cases of resistent infections or septicemia, when granulocyte values were under 100/mm^3.

All blood products were irradiated in vitro with 1500 rad prior to transfusion for 6 weeks from the beginning of conditioning.

RESULTS

No patient died of conditioning toxicity. Four patients out of 14 died within 53-270 days after ALG and marrow infusion of marrow insufficiency with septicemia and hemorrhage. One patient is too early for evaluation.

The pattern of reconstitution of the 6 long-term survivors who have been followed long enough to be reasonably certain of the stability of their remission is shown in Figure 1 (5 patients 1 year and more after ALG + BM, 1 patient 6 months after remission). Three further patients are not recorded in this figure: 2 of them have now achieved a good remission and the 3rd continues to require platelet transfusions.

The time interval between ALG + BM and the moment where the criteria for SAA were not fulfilled anymore is recorded here. By now all these patients have achieved complete remissions. Most patients needed from 1 to 4 months before showing clearcut signs of reconstitution. Reticulocytes and granulocytes were seen first. Platelets came later. Hemo-

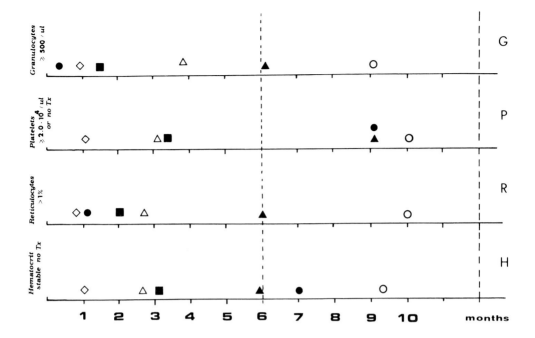

Fig. 1. Time interval between ALG + BM and the moment where the criteria of aplastic anemia were not fulfilled anymore. Symbols represent the different patients.

globin stabilized relatively late and all these patients showed initially signs of very ineffective erythropoiesis with distinct dyserythropoietic features in the bone marrow.

Three patients recovered 6-10 months only after ALG and bone marrow, so that the relation to treatment appears somewhat doubtful.

The course of such a patient with late recovery is shown in Figure 2. After ALG + BM the peripheral blood showed a transient amelioration of the reticulocytes without correction of the anemia. Nine months later the values suddenly ameliorated and the blood picture normalized. Three months before, androgens, which were stopped prior to ALG because the patient was refractory to them, were started again.

Figure 3 showed the same phenomenon in a second patient. He came into remission only 3 months after restarting on androgens, having been refractory to them prior to ALG + BM. Both patients are still androgen dependent. They both need about 10 mg oxymetholone on alternate days. The first patient was documented twice to experience relapse after androgen withdrawal. Restarting was followed by complete restoration in about 6 weeks. Considering the time interval between treatment and reconstitution corrected for androgen beginning after ALG (Fig. 4), all our long-term survivors recovered a sufficient marrow function between 1 and 4½ months after ALG + BM, as did the 2 later patients not

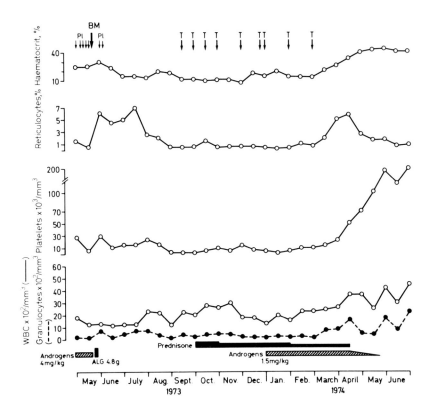

Fig. 2. Hematological course of a patient with late recovery (C.J-L. 1961).

recorded here.

Almost complete reconstitution followed the phase of self-sustaining marrow function with low counts.

Considering further the patients of our series who died we find that none of them had androgens after ALG + BM, because to that time they were considered as refractory and we did not recognize the value of androgens after immunosuppression with ALG.

Figure 5 showed the survival curve of our 13 patients. The overall survival is 69%. If we consider only the patients who received androgens after ALG + BM we have a survival of 100%. Eight of these 9 patients are now off transfusion with self-sustaining hemopoiesis and have virtually complete reconstitutions. The 9th patient has a good reconstitution of the granulocytes and of the erythrocytes but still needs platelet support.

Figure 6 shows the latest granulocyte and platelet values of all the patients. Most patients have now granulocytes over 1000/mm^3 and platelets over 50,000/mm^3. They have self-sustaining erythropoiesis.

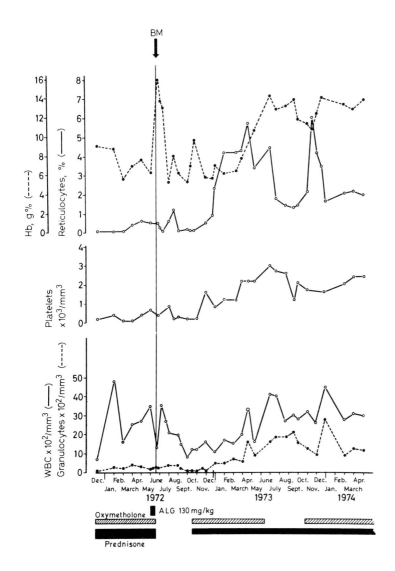

Fig. 3. Hematological course of a second patient with late recovery (H.H. 1964).

DISCUSSION

In our patients there is a clear relation between success and androgen therapy after ALG conditioning and bone marrow infusion, even if the patient was refractory to androgens prior to ALG.

The reason for this is not clear but does not seem to be depending on the kind of androgen used (3 patients had oxymetholone, 3 norethandrolone). One possibility could be some kind of further immunosuppression by a side effect of

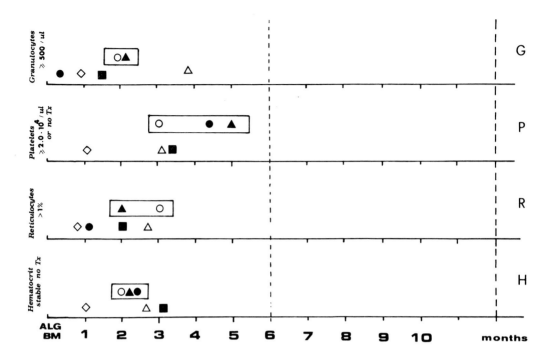

Fig. 4. Time interval between ALG + BM and beginning of reconstitution corrected for restarting on androgens after marrow infusion. Symbols in frames represent patients who were restarted on androgens late and had a 'late recovery'.

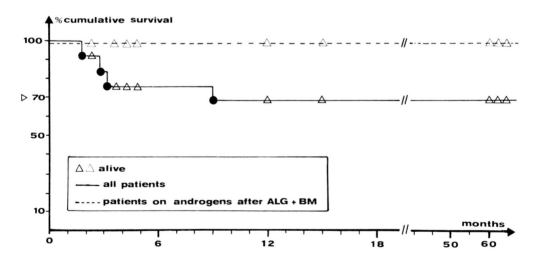

Fig. 5. Survival curves of the 13 evaluable patients. Open symbols represent living patients. The dotted curve represents survival of the patients having been restarted on androgens after marrow infusion. The other curve represents the overall survival.

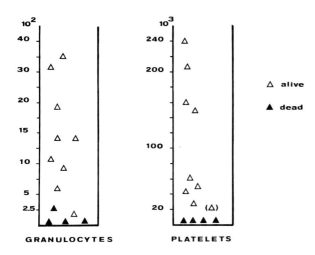

Fig. 6. Latest hematological counts of the 13 evaluable patients. Open symbols represent living patients.

androgens (3). It is also possible that after immunosuppression more stem cells are produced which may respond to androgens.

The second fact which seems very important is the time factor, i.e. the time needed to get a reconstitution after ALG + BM. It is quite different from BMT after cyclophosphamide conditioning (4,5). Autologous reconstitution takes more time than hemopoietic engraftment after a take of matched marrow.

The median time in our patients is about 3 months. Therefore, once ALG is given, optimal supportive care should be given as long as needed in order to provide enough time for a satisfactory evaluation.

We feel that most patients with SAA may experience autologous reconstitution if they are followed and supported in centers with optimal supportive care facilities. One more evidence for that is the fact that even patients after rejection of matched marrow after cyclophosphamide may achieve autologous reconstitution 3-4 months later, provided optimal supportive care is available (6,7). We have now seen 3 such patients out of 5 who rejected matched marrow in the 12 we grafted after cyclophosphamide conditioning. These 3 patients now have a self-sustaining hemopoiesis with only residual thrombocytopenia between 30,000 and 70,000/mm^3, as do some patients after ALG + BM. They all have a normal life.

REFERENCES

1. Speck, B., Cornu, P., Sartorius, J., Nissen, C., Groff, P., Burri, H.P. and Jeannet, M. (1978): Immunologic aspects of aplasia. Transplant. Proc., 10, 131-134.
2. Speck, B., Gluckman, E., Haak, H.L. and Van Rood, J.J. (1977): Treatment of aplastic anemia by antilymphocyte globulin with and without allogeneic bone marrow infusions. Lancet, 2, 1145-1148.

3. Frey-Wettstein, M. and Craddock, C.G. (1970): Testosterone-induced depletion of thymus and marrow lymphocytes as related to lympho-poiesis and hematopoiesis. Blood, 35, 257-271.
4. Thomas, E.D., Storb, R., Clift, R.A., Fefer, A., Johnson, F.L., Neiman, P.E., Lerner, K.G., Glucksberg, H. and Buckner, C.D. (1975): Bone marrow transplantation (Parts I and II). New Engl. J. Med., 292, 832-843 and 895-902.
5. Storb, R., Thomas, E.D., Weiden, P.L., Buckner, C.D., Clift, R.A., Fefer, A., Goodell, B.W., Johnson, F.L., Neiman, P.E., Sanders, J.E. and Singer, J. (1978): One-hundred-ten patients with aplastic anemia treated by marrow transplantation in Seattle. Transplant. Proc., 10, 135-140.
6. Thomas, E.D., Storb, R., Giblett, E.R., Longpre, B., Weiden, P.L., Fefer, A., Witherspoon, R., Clift, R.A. and Buckner, C.D. (1976): Recovery from aplastic anemia following attempted marrow transplanta-tion. Exp. Hematol., 4, 97-102.
7. Speck, B., Cornu, P., Jeannet, M., Nissen, C., Burri, H.P., Groff, P., Nagel, G.A. and Buckner, C.D. (1976): Autologous marrow recovery following allogeneic marrow transplantation in a patient with severe aplastic anemia. Exp. Hematol., 4, 131-137.

SEVERE APLASTIC ANAEMIA IN ADULTS

HISTOLOGICAL OBSERVATIONS IN 13 PATIENTS UNDER ATG TREATMENT

J. te Velde[1], H.L. Haak[2,3], F.E. Zwaan[2,3] and P.J. Spaander[1,3]

[1]Departments of Pathology and [2]Haematology, University Medical Centre and the [3]J.A. Cohen Institute for Radiopathology and Irradiation Protection, Leiden, The Netherlands

SUMMARY

A report on 13 adult patients with severe aplastic anaemia, treated with anti-thymocyte globulin (ATG). Pre- and post-therapy marrow trephine biopsy specimens were embedded in methyl-methacrylate and graded according to the amount and distribution of the inflammatory infiltrate, as described previously. This grading system has been shown to correlate with survival in conventionally treated patients. The additional value of ATG applied to these ATG-treated patients and measured in terms of survival seemed small: 3 patients improved, 2 deteriorated. The 3 responders all belonged to the group of patients with an unfavourable prognosis according to the histological grading. No effect or a reversed effect of ATG was observed in the patients with a favourable prognosis. These observations support our previous findings that aplastic anaemia is a heterogeneous group of disorders, probably partly caused by a destructive autoimmune reaction and partly caused by primary stem cell defect with secondary inflammatory reactions. Before treatment is started the distinction between these subgroups of aplastic anaemia might be made with the help of high quality sections from bone marrow biopsies. Bone marrow histology may help to select those patients for ATG who may respond to immunosuppressive therapy. This would avoid unwanted side effects of such treatment in those who probably will not respond and who may have a good survival under conventional care.

In the Leiden University Hospital, the diagnosis of aplastic anaemia is restricted to patients who present themselves with severe cytopenia of 3 cell lines and a complete or almost complete disappearance of haematopoiesis from the bone marrow. Such patients show no evidence of a deficiency, a metabolic or storage disease or a known or suspected malignancy. In the past 5 years, patients have been studied according to an extensive protocol, including repeated bone marrow trephine biopsies. Biopsy specimens are embedded in plastic to obtain sufficiently high quality sections for histological study of the residual haematopoiesis and the determination of the type and extent of the inflammatory infiltrate (1,2). In retrospective studies, a prognostic significance of the inflammatory infiltrate in the marrow

has been reported. In conventionally treated patients a correlation was found between survival for more than 6 months
and the amount and distribution of the inflammatory infiltrate (2,3). In these studies, as well as in studies involving simultaneous in vitro bone marrow cultures, it seemed
likely that aplastic anaemia was not a single disease entity,
but rather a heterogeneous group of disorders with bone
marrow failure that was not caused by such diseases (excluded by definition) as deficiency, malignancy, etc. (4).
Among our aplastic anaemic adult patients, some seemed to
suffer from an autodestructive immune reaction associated
with or caused by a subpopulation of T cells; other patients
suffered from a primary stem cell defect with a secondary
inflammatory reaction in the marrow. It seemed as if in
severe aplastic anaemia in adults, the differences in aetiol-
ogy were also reflected in differences in the distribution
of the inflammatory infiltrate throughout the marrow.

In our prospective studies on the effect of different
therapeutic regimens in aplastic anaemia in adults, bone
marrow biopsies were performed at regular intervals to esti-
mate the changes in the haematopoiesis and the inflammatory
reaction. This report deals with the histological and clinical findings before and after treatment with anti-thymocyte
globulin (ATG).

METHODS AND MATERIALS

Thirteen patients with severe aplastic anaemia were treated
with ATG between 1974 and 1978. On diagnosing of patients
all had severe anaemia with reticulocytopenia, and granulocyte and thrombocyte counts were below 0.5 and 20 x 10^9/L
respectively. Pretreatment biopsy specimens of patients
with at least 30 mm^2 of bone and bone marrow surface area
in histological sections showed that haematopoiesis was
completely or almost completely absent. On diagnosis, no
evidence was found for the presence of a malignancy, deficiency, metabolic or storage disease, using an extensive
protocol for patient evaluation.

The patients were treated with rabbit ATG in doses of
3 to 5 mg/kg body weight daily for 4 days. In 5 patients
allogeneic bone marrow was transfused after the last dose
of ATG, as described before (5). In no patient was a take
established. The clinical effect of treatment was considered
good if, after an initial further drop of cell counts, the
peripheral blood picture improved within the next weeks to
months with abolishment of the need for transfusions. Any
improvement occurring over a very long period as has been
seen in some patients, has not been attributed to the ATG
treatment because similar partial remissions have also been
observed under conventional treatment. Furthermore, in the
absence of definite recovery following ATG treatment alone,
androgen therapy was usually given to patients.

Bone marrow trephine biopsy specimens were obtained by
trephine, using Burkhardt's or Jamshidi's needle. The tissue

cylinders were embedded in methyl methacrylate, cut at 2 microns and stained as described elsewhere (1). Biopsy specimens were taken at various intervals according to protocol, viz. at the time of referral or diagnosis, before treatment and after treatment at day 2, after 2 and 4 weeks, after 3, 6 and 12 months, and in long-term survivors at irregular intervals.

The histological sections were reviewed without knowledge of the patient's name or course of disease. Only those specimens containing at least 30 mm of bone and bone marrow in the sections were evaluated.

The inflammatory infiltrate was described as mixed when lymphocytes, plasma cells, histiocytic macrophages and mast cells were present in about equal amounts. When either cell type was conspicuously present or dominant it was described as mixed/lymphocytic or as plasmocellular, etc. The amount of infiltrate was estimated as slightly or markedly increased. In markedly increased amounts of infiltrate, it was determined whether this increase was present in all marrow fields. On this basis each specimen was graded as follows:

Grade   I: slightly increased infiltrate
Grade   II: markedly increased infiltrate that spared some areas of fatty and/or haematopoietic marrow
Grade III: markedly increased infiltrate in all marrow areas

Further details and illustrations have been published by Te Velde et al. (2,3,4).

RESULTS

Histology

Pretreatment biopsy specimens all showed a complete or almost complete absence of haematopoiesis and a markedly increased inflammatory infiltrate. In 6 patients specimens were scored as Grade II, in 7 patients as Grade III. The composition of infiltrates is given in Tables 1 and 2. Necrosis of the microcirculation was hardly present. Only focal oedema was found. Even the slightest increase of   s fibres was absent.

By 2 days after ATG infusion, severe changes could be observed. Lymphocytes had usually disappeared although not in all patients. Vascular disarrangement with massive oedema and a dense plasmocellular histiocytic infiltrate could be found in a few patients, while in others hardly any change could be discerned.

At 2 weeks and later, a similar diversity between the patients was present. Only in 3 patients was a striking reduction of the infiltrate observed together with a reappearance of normal haematopoiesis. In 1 patient, however, the specimen taken after 3 months showed epitheloid granuloma, as in sarcoidosis. In 4 other survivors, however, no

TABLE 1. Grade II specimens, histology, effect of ATG, and survival

| Patient | Composition of the infiltrate | | Histological grade after ATG | Clinical effect and survival for more than 6 months |
	Before ATG	After ATG		
vW	ly	ly -	unchanged II	short-term improvement, relapse, alive
dW	ly	ly -	unchanged II	no effect, alive
MB[x]	mixed	ly +	unchanged II	no effect, alive
PT[x]	mixed	mixed	increase to III	no effect, died after 2nd course of ATG
vdZ	mixed/ly	ly -	unchanged II	died 4 weeks after ATG
Ve	mixed			died during ATG treatment

[x]Patients receiving allogeneic bone marrow during ATG treatment. ly = predominantly lymphocytic infiltrate. plasmoc = predominantly plasmocellular infiltrate. mixed = infiltrate consisting of lymphocytes, plasma cells, histiocytes and mast cells without predominance of either type of cell. mixed/ly = mixed infiltrate with conspicuous amounts of lymphocytes. ly - = decrease of the relative amount of lymphocytes, compared to the pretreatment biopsy specimen. ly + = increase of the relative amount of lymphocytes, compared with the pretreatment biopsy specimen.

TABLE 2. Grade III specimens, histology, effect of ATG, and survival

| Patient | Composition of the infiltrate | | Histological grade after ATG | Clinical effect and survival for more than 6 months |
	Before ATG	After ATG		
JJ[x]	ly	ly -	decrease to I	good effect, alive
GN	ly	ly -	decrease to I	good effect, alive
Kr	mixed/ly	ly -	decrease to II	good effect, alive
RM[x]	mixed	ly +	decrease after 18 months	no effect, slow improvement starting after 1 year
Ze	plasmoc	plasmoc	unchanged III	no effect, died after 2nd course of ATG
vE	mixed/ly	ly -		died within 2 weeks
BK	mixed/ly	ly -		died within 2 weeks

For explanation, see Note under Table 1.

reduction was found within the first year, and in 2 patients lymphocytes surprisingly became the dominant cell type in the infiltrate.

Histological grading, effect of ATG and survival

From earlier studies it had appeared that the distinction between patients in Grades II and III could be used to distinguish survivors from patients with a very poor prognosis, and also for making a subdivision between different types of aplastic anaemia. Therefore, we divided our ATG-treated patients according to our grading system (Tables 1 and 2). Seven out of 13 patients survived 6 to 45 months; 3 had initially been graded II, 4 as Grade III. Again, there is a marked difference between both grades since from the 3 survivors in Grade II only 1 patient showed some improvement in blood cell counts, which could be ascribed to ATG. However, the effect was very weak and of short duration. The 3 patients showing a rapid improvement of blood cell values had all been graded as Grade III. One Grade III patient did not show a similar response. Her values started to rise very slowly after 1 year and after 1.5 years her grading was changed because of the distribution throughout the marrow, rather than because of a change in the amount of infiltrate. Six patients have died. Three patients had been graded as Grade II, which is associated with long-term survival under conventional treatment. One Grade II patient died during ATG treatment due to a hypersensitivity reaction. The second patient was known to have a stable pancytopenia without infectious complications for several years before ATG treatment. Shortly after the infusions, herpes lesions appeared; they became infected and formed the 'porte d'entrée' for uncontrollable septicaemia, leading to death. In both patients, the effect of ATG treatment was considered negative rather than positive (Table 3). In Grade II patients (Table 1) 1 more patient died. He was treated with 2 courses of ATG without any clinical effect. In the last weeks, his histological grade progressed to Grade III and he died of haemorrhage and infection 4 weeks afterwards. Three patients of Grade III have died (Table 2). Two patients had received ATG in a last effort to alleviate the aplasia, failing suitable bone marrow transplant donors. Both patients

TABLE 3. Clinical effect of ATG

	Positive	None	Negative	No time to evaluate
Grade II	–	4 (3)	2 (0)	–
Grade III	3 (3)	2 (1)	–	2 (0)

In parentheses, patients surviving 6 months.

were severely infected and died of septicaemia within 2 weeks. In both, the biopsy specimens at day 2 showed a disappearance of the lymphocytes and dense oedema with vascular disarrangement. This was also observed in the responding patients, but the clinical effect of ATG could not be evaluated. The 3rd Grade III patient, dying 3 months after a second course of ATG, did not show any clinical effect or histological change in grade or composition of the infiltrate.

DISCUSSION

Aplastic anaemia is the name for a variety of disorders, having in common the absence of haematopoiesis at the time of diagnosis and the absence of certain diseases, known to be associated with marrow insufficiency, such as malignancies, deficiencies, etc. A primary stem cell defect is one of the causes of aplastic anaemia and supplementation of stem cells from identical twins can be used to restore the marrow functions, but stem cells cannot be maintained in vitro. However, recovery of the marrow function is also observed after immunosuppressive treatment with or without bone marrow transplantation. This observation strengthened the hypothesis that some form of immune disorder in the marrow might be the cause of aplastic anaemia. Both hypotheses can be sustained by observations on different patients. This most likely indicates that at least one or both mechanisms can be held responsible for the onset of the aplasia. In retrospective studies on the effectiveness of stem cell transfusions or immunosuppressive regimens, one should be able to distinguish between at least 2 different groups of aplastic anaemic patients. If the effect of any form of treatment is evaluated in survival times, then one should also know the change for survival under conventional supportive care in the individual patient and the additional risk of the therapy.

   In our earlier studies, we have proposed a subdivision between patients on the basis of histological differences in amount and distribution of the inflammatory infiltrate in their marrow biopsy specimens. It appeared that patients with a weak infiltrate were usually in clinical remission. But patients with severe aplastic anaemia and having a strong infiltrate, could be distinguished from patients with a strong infiltrate in all marrow fields (Grade III) and patients with a strong infiltrate sparing some marrow fields (Grade II). Under conventional treatment, Grade III was associated with death within 6 months after biopsy, while Grade II patients with equally severe aplasia came into remission and survived for longer periods, although complete normalization of the marrow function was not observed (2,3). In combined histological and in vitro culture studies (4), we speculated whether this distinction also correlated with differences in pathogenesis. The number of patients studied was small, due to the rarity of the disease. The observations discussed here, however, still seem to be consistent with our earlier findings.

In the 13 patients in this series, immunosuppression by ATG induced a clinical remission in 3 patients, each having been scored as Grade III before treatment. This clinical reaction was accompanied by a remarkable reaction of the infiltrate in the marrow biopsy specimens. This clinical and histological reaction was not observed in Grade II patients. In the group of Grade III patients, 2 died before any clinical effect could be observed. Two further patients did not respond clearly to the treatment given. Neither of the patients had conspicuous amounts of lymphocytes in their pretreatment biopsy specimens. In the 1 survivor, lymphocytes appeared after 18 months in a period of slow recovery. These incidental observations in a minority of the patients should be repeated, before concluding that the histological differences seen in the composition of the infiltrate are associated with differences in pathogenesis of the aplasia. One may expect that a predominantly plasmo-cellular infiltrate interferes in a different manner with the haematopoiesis than an infiltrate mainly composed of T cell subpopulations (1). However, in the non-responding Grade II patients, the composition of the infiltrate was about the same as in the responding Grade III patients, the only difference being the distribution of the infiltrate throughout the marrow. This could be explained by the possibility that in aplastic anaemia different inflammatory cell types play different roles in the development of marrow insufficiency, and that the importance of their role cannot be deduced from their mere presence. It seems, however, that their dissemination throughout the marrow may give a clue about the primary role they play. In the disseminated lymphocyte-rich Grade III patients, removal of the infiltrate by ATG induced a restoration of the marrow function, while in the non-disseminated Grade II patients the same treatment did not show the same effect, possibly because the presence of the infiltrate was secondary, for example, to a primary stem cell defect.

In terms of survival, the results of this small series are comparable to those of bone marrow transplantation: 6 of 13 patients survive for 6 to 45 months. However, if we are right in assuming that the Grade II patients already had a favourable prognosis, one might have expected about an equal number of survivors under conventional care alone: 6 out of 13. Of the 7 patients with a poor prognosis (Grade III), 3 clearly benefitted from the ATG treatment, while 2 Grade II patients had their lives shortened by the same treatment.

The conclusion must be reached that overall the value of ATG has not been convincingly demonstrated in terms of survival. Yet it changed the course of the disease in 3 out of the 7 patients with a very poor prognosis. If we can select either those patients who will not respond or even those who may only suffer from ill side effects, then ATG can be shown to be a valuable way of treatment in aplastic anaemia. This selection procedure is obviously also of great importance in prospective trials. From our observations it seems that well-prepared bone marrow biopsy sections do help in this selection. Thus, bone marrow histology can contribute not only in making the diagnosis, but probably in assessing the prognosis, the choice of therapy and in the evaluation of the effect of various ways of treatment.

REFERENCES

1. Te Velde, J., Burkhardt, R., Kleiverda, K., Leenheers-Binnendijk, L. and Sommerfeld, W. (1977): Methyl-methacrylate as an embedding medium in histopathology. Histopathology, 1, 319-330.
2. Te Velde, J. and Haak, H.L. (1977): Aplastic anaemia. Histological investigation of methacrylate embedded bone marrow biopsy specimens. Brit. J. Haemat., 35, 61-69.
3. Te Velde, J. and Haak, H.L. (1978):Aplastic anaemia in adults. Further evidence for the significance of the inflammatory infiltrate in methacrylate embedded bone marrow biopsy specimens. Bibl. haemat. (Basel), 45, 96-102.
4. Haak, H.L., Goselink, H.M., Veenhof, W., Pellinkhof-Stadelman, S., Kleiverda, J.K. and Te Velde, J. (1977): Acquired aplastic anaemia in adults. Histological and CFU studies in transplanted and non-transplanted patients. Scand. J. Haemat., 19, 159-171.
5. Speck, B., Gluckman, E., Haak, H.L. and Van Rood, J.J. (1978): Treatment of aplastic anaemia by antilymphocyte globulin with or without marrow infusion. Clin. in Haemat., 7, 611.

BONE MARROW MORPHOLOGY AFTER MARROW TRANSPLANTATION

WITH SPECIAL REFERENCE TO ERYTHROBLASTIC ISLANDS AND
MACROPHAGIC REACTIONS

Alberto Marmont

Division of Hematology and Clinical Immunology, Ospedale
Regionale S. Martino, Genova, Italy

SUMMARY

The dynamic morphology of the bone marrow (BM) has been studied in 10
patients who underwent bone marrow transplantation (BMT) for severe
aplastic anemia (SAA) and acute myeloid leukemia (AML). Of 7 cases of
SAA 4 were from histocompatible and 3 were from haploid donors. The
medullary material was obtained by aspiration, but treated so as to
preserve the BM architecture. Postvital preparations were particularly
useful.
     In patients with SAA, the BM before transplantation showed a
typical 'aplastic granuloma' composed of macrophages, mast cells, lymphocytes and plasmacytes; after BMT, repopulation always started at the
periphery of the granulomata, but never in the midst of same. Granulocytic repopulations preceded erythropoiesis. The latter always took
place by way of typical erythroblastic islands; the number of erythroblasts suggested possible derivations both from BFU-Es and CFU-Es.
Marked but transitory dyserythropoietic aspects were found in 1 case.
     Both in SAA and in AML, but more so in the latter, a marked
macrophagic hyperplasia could be found in the earlier stages after
BMT. 'Activated' and phagocytosing macrophages were present; these last
engulfing hemoglobin-derived granules and nucleated cells. This last
category was foremost in rejection episodes.

Although the number of allogeneic BMTs is quite high, little
attention has been given to dynamic BM morphology after
transplantation. One of the original findings was that
typical erythroblastic islands appeared in the regenerating
and expanding allogeneic BM (1,2). Characteristic dyserythropoietic features could be observed in an early and transitional stage in 1 case (1,2), apart from the frequent
existence of a ring of early reticulocytes adhering to the
external erythroblast layers (1,2), as already described in
all types of stimulated erythropoiesis (3). Discrete erythroid, myeloid and mixed megakaryocytic-erythroid colonies
were also found in BM histologic sections after successful
transplantation by Cline et al.(4).
     The morphological study presented here, besides extend-
ing previous observations (1,2), gives additional information concerning the physiopathology of transplantation,

neohemopoiesis and, hopefully, some indications for a better therapeutic management.

MATERIAL AND METHODS

Ten BMTs have been performed to date at our Institution, 7 of which were from wholly histocompatible and 3 from haploidentical donors. A summary of this clinical material is given in Table 1.

TABLE 1

Diseases	Cases	ABO incomp.(major)	Take	Rejection	GVH	Survival
SAA	7	2^x	4^{xx}	2$^'$	2$^"$	4$^+$
AML	3	2^x	3	-		-

^{x}Total plasma exchange and Witebsky's substance. ^{xx}Phenotypic and cytogenetic switches; no take with 2 haploidentical donors. $^'$One lethal. $^"$All resolved with massive bolus corticotherapy and/or ALG. $^+$>780, >210, >160, >100, >40, >30, 34 days.

    Sternal and posterior iliac crest BM was obtained by conventional aspirations; the aspirates were anticoagulated and firmly but gently spread on the slides. No 'smears' of medullary blood were made. These dried preparations were stained by Romanowsky stains (generally May-Grünwald-Giemsa), Perls's stain for iron and various cytochemical methods. In addition, postvital (5) preparations of medullary droplets were made utilising brilliant cresyl blue, new methylene blue^x and cresyl violet, and acridine orange. The latter combined with fluorescence microscopy as already described elsewhere (2,3).

RESULTS

While the appearance of BM in AML transplantation will not be described here, one specific aspect in SAA will be given. Postvital preparations were especially consistent in showing aggregates of reticulum cells, activated macrophages (see below), mast cells and, to a lesser degree, plasmacytes and lymphocytes, in addition to hemopoietic cells. These aggregates were defined as 'aplastic granulomata'.
    After transplantation, no discrete aggregates could be found in SAA until at least 2 weeks after BMT, after which a gradual progress to cellularity was made, with the appearance of cells at about 4 weeks. Repopulation never took place in the midst of aplastic granulomata, but al-

^{x}'Testsimplets' Boehringer.

20

ways at the periphery of same. Later, the granulomata disappeared completely, and the BM assumed a parenchymal cellularity. In AML aggregates could still be found during the first 2 weeks after BMT, but they were composed of severely damaged (and presumably dying out) leukemic cells and a rapidly increasing population of macrophages.

No primitive looking, totally undifferentiated cells could be observed at any time, even when early hypocellular aspirates were examined on smears prepared by the Shandon cytocentrifuge. On these preparations, markedly immature cells with basophilic cytoplasm rich in primary azurophilic granules (early promyelocytes; 'myeloblasts' according to Ferrata-Bessis (4)), were the earliest precursors which could be identified by light microscopy. Except in 1 case

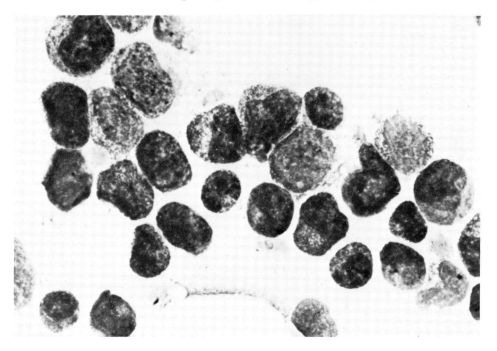

Fig. 1. Early granulocytoblastic colony. Promyelocytes and myelocytes being dominant.

granulocytopoiesis always preceded erythropoiesis, paralleling the appearance of granulocytes in the blood, 10-15 days before reticulocytes. Discrete granulocytoblastic aggregates were often observed, both of a synchronous and asynchronous character.

The erythroblastic repopulation invariably took place as erythroblastic islands. These were generally synchronous, i.e., composed of cells exhibiting the same degree of

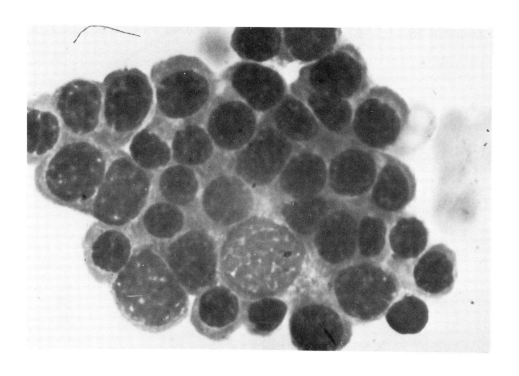

Fig. 2. A typical erythroblastic island.

maturation, basophilic, polychromatic or orthochromatic; non-synchronous islands were considerably more rare. This finding was prominent in all patients, whether transplanted for SAA or AL. It could be observed with all methods but especially so on the fresh, postvital preparations; even with the smearing technique, when not performed too clumsily, elongated islands could still be recognized.

The number of single erythroblasts contained in any single island was variable, but generally high, between 50 and 400, while early synchronous islands (presumably basophilic) were not surrounded by reticulocytes. These were plentiful around the more mature ones, and were sometimes interspersed in them. While in our first case, nuclear budding, fragmentation and other dyserythropoietic aspects were prominent, similar changes were much less pronounced in the other cases. Only in 1 case of AML, who died of interstitial pneumonia on day +73, did the last BM aspirate (+70) show extreme dyserythropoiesis, especially in the orthochromatic stages, a feature which had been completely absent in all the former aspirates. This patient had been receiving 400 mg of trimethoprim and 4 g of sulfamethoxazole daily for 10 days.

A marked macrophagic hyperplasia could be observed in all these marrows. However, some morphologic diversities

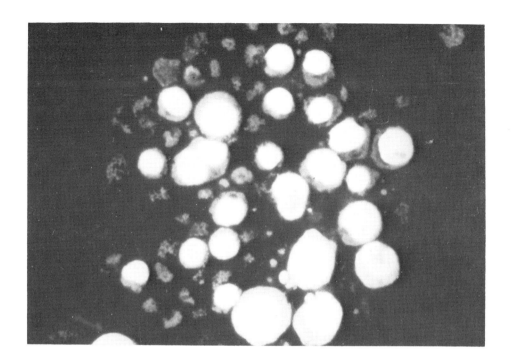

Fig. 3. Erythroblastic islands seen by fluorescence microscopy after fluorochromization with acridine orange. The adherent reticulocytes are clearly visible.

were seen with a certain regularity, so that 4 subtypes could be recognized.
1.   Type I was composed of spread-out, clasmatocytic, macrophages. They were generally non-phagocytic, or containing a few scarce darkish granules. This was the most frequent subtype.
2.   Type II macrophages were mainly phagocytic, containing Hb-derived granules, which were intensely Perls positive. They also phagocytosed erythrocytes. They were found to be prominent in ABO major incompatibilities, irrespective of the primitive SAA or AML nature of the disease.
3.   Type III macrophages were foamy cells. They were found especially in AML after chemotherapy and TBI, and formed an additional population to that seen in AML after heavy chemotherapy. In 1 case, at a defined time point they contributed up to 40% of the total BM cellularity.
4.   Type IV macrophages phagocytosed nucleated cells, whether erythroblasts or granulocytoblasts or both. The phagocytosed cells were apparently frequently damaged. The appearance of these macrophages was closely similar to those found in histocytic medullary reticulosis (malignant histiocytosis). This subtype was most frequent in the

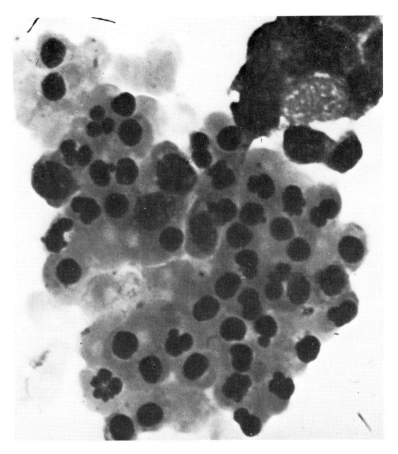

Fig. 4. A typical orthochromatic erythroblastic island from Case 1 displaying marked dyserythropoiesis. Nuclear budding and fragmentation are evident.

rejection episodes.

Although these subtypes could be distinguished, an admixture of all types was often present. In any case, the most marked macrophagic hyperplasia was found in the first week after BMT for AML, while nucleated cell phagocytosis, though occurring in all situations, was really prominent in the rejection episodes, where it was associated with lymphocytosis, plasmacytosis and the presence of transformed lymphocytes.

DISCUSSION

Although histology is currently undergoing a renaissance in the morphologic study of SAA (6,7) and BMT (4), the advantages of proper cytomorphology should not be overlooked, nor the method summarily discarded. One of the chief reasons for the devaluation of aspiration cytomorphology is the

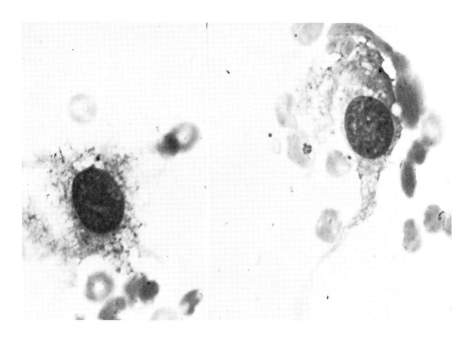

Fig. 5. Activated macrophages. Streaming, lacy cytoplasmic projection
are clearly visible.

habit of performing smears with medullary blood, and studying single cells separately. However, these are only equiv-
alents of peripheral blood smears, and fail to give information on BM cellularity and architecture. Aggregate
imprinting, careful spreading (not smearing) and the observation of postvital preparations of marrow particles
enables not only single cell identification (at best only
approximate in histologic sections), but the recognition
of·special features such as dyserythropoiesis, reticulo-
cytosis all around erythroblastic islands, macrophage
diversity and activation, 'aplastic granuloma' and other
aspects.
      Before discussing these morphologic findings I wish to
make a short comment on the repopulation of the BM by the
migrating allogeneic stem cells, a phenomenon generically
referred to as homing (8) or nostocytosis (5). Pluripotent
stem cells must first be fixed in the BM sinusoids by a
preferential trapping mechanism, but then migration through
the wall of the vascular sinuses must be postulated. The
BM microenvironment appears to be so constructed as to
allow the entry and exit of stem cells (9), but, until more
is known about their mobility, which is generally regarded
as scarce, little can be said concerning this fascinating

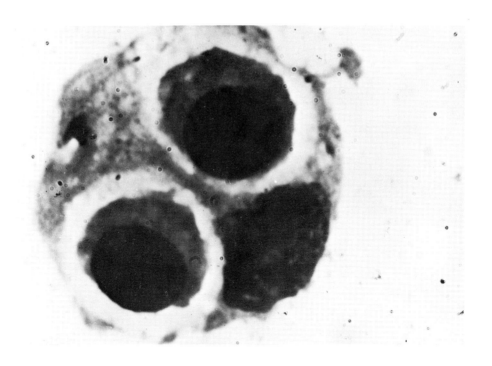

Fig. 6. Macrophage ingesting two apparently undamaged erythroblasts during a rejection episode.

phenomenon of BM reseeding. An active role for the perisinal adventitial cells in the regulation of transmural cell migration from the marrow has been demonstrated by Tavassoli (10), and it is quite possible that a cooperation between adventitial and reticular cells may be operative in this sort of 'reversed' diapedesis. This particular micro-environment could obviate the presumptive greater rigidity of the highly immature stem cells; on the other hand, it is composed of relatively chemo- and radioresistant cells. Do stem cells from nonanemic littermates of Steel mice remain in the marrow sinusoids and not penetrate the extrasinus-oidal space? Hopefully this point could be elucidated by some capable experimentalist.

The presence of the 'aplastic granulomata' on post-vital preparations was one of the most striking findings in SAA. They are entirely superimposable with the 'inflammatory infiltrate' which has been recently described in histologi-cal sections by Te Velde and Haak (6); I have likewise found a clear correlation between this finding and the severity of the disease. It is also of note that hematologic repopulation, whether after bona fide BMT after treatment with massive bolus corticotherapy, ALG, ALG plus haploid BMT and the like, always took place out of the granulomata and never in their midst. It is proposed that the 'aplastic

26

granuloma' takes an active part in the pathogenesis of SAA, and that its demonstration by supravital aspiration technique is practically equivalent - even if not in durable specimens - to histologic sections.

The earliest progenitors I have been able to observe after BMT were differentiated: early promyelocytes and pro-erythroblasts. 'Undifferentiated' colonies such as those observed by Cline et al. (4) were never seen. However, their identification in histologic sections appears questionable.

By far the most frequent findings were the erythroblastic and reticulocytopoietic islands. This was true both in SAA and in AML after BMT, as well as in SAA treated with and responding to ALG. The phenomenon was identical to the one observed in erythroblastic repopulation in pure red cell aplasia after immunosuppressive treatment (11,12). When the erythroblastic islands were synchronous, they were superimposable on the erythroid amplification phenomenon recently described in the rat (13). In the non-synchronous islands, each erythroblastic layer appeared to be of the same degree of maturation (14). The often extremely high (200) or moderate (50) number of erythroblasts for each island may well have corresponded to the BFU-E or CFU-E nature of the progenitor cell.

Dyserythropoiesis was observed in 2 cases. In the first, a case of SAA fully described elsewhere (1,2), its transient character made us postulate a stress or para-physiologic phenomenon. The finding of extreme orthochromatic dyserythropoiesis on day +70 after BMT in a patient dying with interstitial pneumonia, and in whom there was also some degree of myeloblastic transformation, is perhaps to be regarded as an acquired secondary dyserythropoiesis (15) due to high doses of a combination of trimethoprim and sulfamethoxazole, notoriously capable of inducing folate deficiency.

Macrophagic reactions were constant, and at times quite imposing. The various morphological aspects which have been described are not to be interpreted as a claim to a differentiation in regular subtypes, but rather give an idea of the diversity of macrophagic responses. The spread-out, clasmatocytic macrophages are most probably activated macrophages (16), as seen in the setting of BMT. Macrophages phagocytosing Hb-derived pigments were prominent in ABO major incompatibility, in which isohemoagglutinins had been removed by means of plasma exchanges and absorbed with Witebsky substances, but a certain degree of subclinical hemolysis was still present until the complete blood group switch took place (1,2). However, the most interesting aspect is the macrophagic hyperplasia and phagocytosis in the course of rejection.

Although the presence of macrophages at sites of allo-graft rejection is well established, their presence during BMT has yet to be reported. Alveolar macrophages have been shown to derive from donor monocytic precursors after BMT in man (17), and it is to be regretted that a search for Y bodies in BM macrophages after male-to-female BMT has not been done in our cases. Hopefully, it will be made in future. However, indirect evidence, including chemo- and radioresistance, makes me postulate that all these BM macrophages were of recipient origin; their early appearance in AML after TBI makes the hypothesis of donor derivation untenable.

Regarding their significance, the macrophages could be envisaged as having a primary role in graft destruction, or, alternatively, they could be merely involved in phagocytosis of tissue debris resulting from the cytotoxic activity of another cell type (18). Phagocytosis was prominent, but it must be borne in mind that this may be a late effect (19), the killing effect being mediated by prior cell-to-cell interactions possibly implicating lysosome translocation from the cytotoxic macrophages to the target cells (20). Thus, the question of whether the macrophages appearing in the rejection of transplanted allogenic BM are 'killers' or 'undertakers' remains unsolved (21). Macrophages are prominent in untreated SAA (22), but the demonstration of a probable autoimmune pathogenesis in this disease (23) makes their role, once again, doubtful. Their scavenger role after chemoradiotherapeutic eradication of AML is clear. However, the demonstration that BM may be successfully grafted between unrelated, histocompatible dogs after treatment of the recipient animals with colloidal silica, which destroys macrophages (24), makes the subject worthy of additional investigation.

REFERENCES

1. Marmont, A.M., Damasio, E.E., Bacigalupo, A., Giordano, D., Rossi, E., Reali, G., Gay, A., Dagna-Bricarelli, F., Brema, F., Carella, A.M. and Santini, G. (1977): A to O bone marrow transplantation in severe aplastic anaemia: dynamics of blood group conversion and demonstration of early dyserythropoiesis in the engrafted marrow. Brit. J. Haemat., 36, 511.
2. Marmont, A.M., Avanzi, G., Bacigalupo, A., Brema, F., Carella, A.M., Cerri, R., Damasio, E.E., Dagna-Bricarelli, F., Gay, A., Giordano, D., Piaggio, G., Queirolo, M.A., Raffo, M., Reali, G., Risso, M., Rossi, E., Santini, G. and Van Lint, M.T. (1978): Il trapianto di midollo nella mielopatia globale aplastica. In: Atti XXVI Congr. Soc. It. Ematol., p. 211. Tip. Viscontea, Pavia.
3. Marmont, A.M. and Damasio, E.E. (1962): Fluorescence microscopy in haematology, with special regard to the reticulocytopoietic activity of the so-called erythroblastic nests or islands. In: Proc. 8th Congress Europ. Soc. Haemat., Vol. 1, p. 66. S. Karger, Basel.
4. Cline, M.J., Gale, R.P. and Golde, D.W. (1977): Discrete clusters of hemopoietic cells in the marrow cavity of man after bone marrow transplantation. Blood, 50, 709.
5. Bessis, M. (1976): Réinterprétation des Frottis Sanguins. Masson-Springer, Paris-Berlin.

6. Te Velde, J. and Haak, H.L. (1977): Aplastic anaemia. Histological investigation of methacrylate embedded bone marrow biopsy specimens; correlation with survival after conventional treatment in 15 adult patients. Brit. J. Haemat., 35, 61-69.

7. Duhamel, G., Muratore, R., Bryon, P.A. and Horchowski, N. (1978): Les lésions histologiques de la moëlle dans l'aplasie médullaire. Resultats d'un protocole commun portant sur 261 biopsies. Nouv. Rev. franç. Hémat., 20, 17-32.

8. Weiss, P. and Andres, G. (1952): Experiments on the fate of embryonic cells (chick) disseminated by the vascular route. J. exp. Zool., 121, 449.

9. Metcalf, D. and Moore, M.A.S. (1971): Haemopoietic Cells. North-Holland Publ. Co., Amsterdam-London.

10. Tavassoli, M. (1977): Adaptation of marrow sinus wall to fluctuation in the rate of cell delivery: studies in rabbits after bloodletting. Brit. J. Haemat., 35, 25.

11. Marmont, A.M. (1974): Pure erythroblastopenia or red cell aplasia: an autoimmune disease responding to immunodepressive therapy. In: Present Problems in Haematology, p. 255. Editors: J. Libansky and L. Donner. Excerpta Medica, Amsterdam.

12. Marmont, A.M., Peschle, C., Sanguineti, M. and Condorelli, M. (1975): Pure red cell aplasia (PRCA): response of three patients to cyclophosphamide and/or antilymphocytic globulin (ALG) and demonstration of two types of serum IgG inhibitors to erythropoiesis. Blood, 45, 247.

13. Mize, C., Prenant, M., Pourreau, N. and Bessis, M. (1977): Etude 'in vivo' de l'amplification au cours de l'érythropoièse du rat. Nouv. Rev. franç. Hémat., 18, 627.

14. Le Charpentier, Y. and Prenant, M. (1975): Isolement de l'ilôt érithroblastique. Etude en microscopie optique et électronique à balayage. Nouv. Rev. franç. Hémat., 15, 119.

15. Lewis, S.M. and Verwilghen, R.L. (1977): Dyserythropoiesis: definition, diagnosis and assessment. In: Dyserythropoiesis. Editors: S.M. Lewis and R.L. Verwilghen. Academic Press, London-New York-S. Francisco.

16. Mackanese, G.B. (1970): The mechanism of macrophage activation. In: Infectious Agents and Host Reactions, pp. 61-75. Saunders, Philadelphia.

17. Thomas, E.D., Ramberg, R.E., Sale, G.E., Sparkes, R.S. and Golde, D.W. (1976): Direct evidence for a bone marrow origin of the alveolar macrophage in man. Science, 196, 1016.

18. Jones, B., Jones, T.C. and Roitt, I.M. (1977): Allograft cytotoxicity. Two populations of effector cells detectable by cytolytic and cytostatic assays in vitro. Immunology, 32, 591.

19. Alexander, P. (1977): Macrophages and tumours. Schweiz. med. Wschr., 106, 1345.

20. Bucana, C., Hoyer, L.C., Hobbs, B., Breesman, S., McDaniel, M. and Hanna, M.C. Jr. (1976): Morphological evidence for the translocation of lysosomal organelles from cytotoxic macrophages into the cytoplasm of tumor target cells. Cancer Res., 36, 4444.

21. Marmont, A. (1978): Macrophages in bone marrow transplant reactions. Haematologica, 63, 91.

22. Frisch, B. and Lewis, J.M. (1974): The bone marrow in aplastic anaemia: diagnostic and prognostic features. J. clin. Path, 27, 231.

29

23. Speck, B., Cornu, P., Sartorius, J., Nissen, C., Groff, P., Burri, H.P. and Jeannet, M. (1978): Immunologic aspects of aplasia. Transplant. Proc., 10, 131.

24. Vriesendorp, H.M. and Van Bekkum, D.W.: cited by Calne, R.Y. (1976): Mechanisms in the acceptance of organ grafts. Brit. med. Bull., 32, 107.

THE EFFECT OF ATG ON ABNORMAL MITOGEN STIMULATION IN PATIENTS WITH APLASTIC ANEMIA

L.J.M. Sabbe[1], H.L. Haak[2], B.A. Bradley[1] and J.J. van Rood[1]

[1]Department of Immunohaematology, University Medical Centre, Leiden, and [2]Isolation Ward, J.A. Cohen Institute of Radio-pathology and Radiation Protection, Leiden, The Netherlands

SUMMARY

Seven aplastic anemia patients, treated with anti-thymocyte-globulin (ATG) with or without allogeneic bone marrow infusion, have been tested repeatedly in the lymphocyte transformation test. Five patients had very weak reactions to Pokeweed mitogen and three were hyporesponsive to Concanavalin A before therapy. One patient was tested in a cell mediated lymphocytotoxic assay in which she expressed a very high cytotoxic capacity. This same patient was completely unreactive to a battery of antigens. In all patients all parameters normalized after ATG except in one patient who died 5 months later. These results strengthen the hypothesis of an immune pathogenesis for aplastic anemia.

Together with Dr. E. Gluckman (St Louis, Paris) and Dr. B. Speck (Kantonsspital, Basel) we have recently published a study in which the effect of ATG on the clinical course of severe aplastic anemia was assessed (1). Our conclusions were that:
a. about half of the patients suffering from severe aplastic anemia improved significantly after 4 daily doses of ATG;
b. it was unlikely that this was due to patient selection in the sense that we had selected patients who without ATG treatment would have survived anyhow;
c. it was possible that the ATG removed from the bone marrow T cells interfered with the differentiation of the stem cells. A possibility which is strongly supported by in vitro studies by one of us (2) and others (3).
     To gain a further insight in the mechanism by which ATG corrects the differentiation-blocking effect of T cells in aplastic anemia the in vitro mitogen and antigen response as measured by the lymphocyte transformation test (LTT) was determined. It could be shown that in some of the patients the mitogen and antigen induced LTT was abnormally high or low and that ATG treatment in the majority of the cases studied corrected these abnormalities. One patient was also studied using the cell mediated lympholysis (CML) test. An abnormal high Cr^{51} release was found before ATG, which was normalized after ATG.

MATERIALS AND METHODS

All patients were treated in the Department of Haematology
(head Prof. E.A. Loelinger). The relevant data of these patients is given in Table 1. Follow-up data are shown in
Figure 1. Nos. 1 to 5 correspond with Nos. 1 to 5 of our
previous publication. Lymphocytes were collected before and
at several times after ATG treatment. The mitogen LTT test
and the cell mediated lympholysis test were carried out as
described elsewhere (4,5). Mitogens used were: Phytohemagglutinin (PHA)(Wellcome) at a final dilution of 1/100 and
1/400, Pokeweed mitogen (PWM, Grand Island Biological Company) at the same dilution, and Concanavalin A (Con A, Cal-
biochem. San Diego) at final dilutions of 5 and 20 µg/ml.
As antigens we used Varidase R (Lederle), containing 100,000
IU Streptokinase and 100,000 IU Streptodornase, at final
dilutions of 1/200 and 1/2000, Candida albicans allergic

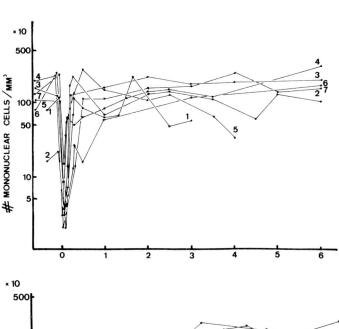

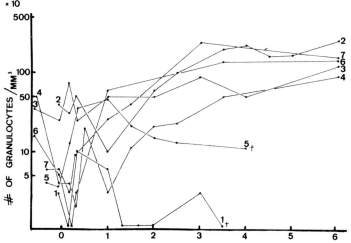

TABLE 1. Hematological values of the patients described at the time of admission

Case	Age	Sex	Reti's $^{0}/_{00}$	Neutro's x10^{-9}/l	Ly x10^{-9}/l	Platelets x10^{-9}/l	Sx	Therapy	Improved
1 (He)	50	F	0	0.15	1.5	10	-	ATG + BM	-
2 (Ji)	14	F	6	0.27	0.1	22	-	ATG + BM	+
3 (Bo)	24	M	120	0.24	1.0	7	40 d	ATG + BM	+
4 (Re)	42	F	0	0.03	0.5	10	50 d	ATG + BM	+
5 (To)	14	M	4	0.04	1.0	3	50 d	ATG + BM	-
6 (KD)	38	F	14	0.16	0.8	7.5	-	ATG	+/-
7 (GN)	30	F	0	0.02	1.3	5	-	ATG	+

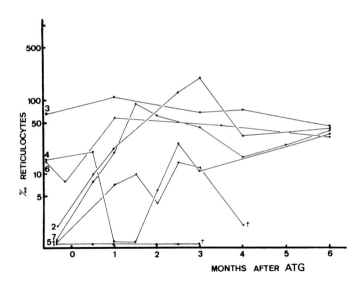

Fig. 1. Evolution of the immunological parameters (a) Response to Concanavalin A. (b) Response to Pokeweed mitogen. (c) Response to Varidase
R all in counts per minute.

extract (Hollister-Stier) diluted 100 and 400 times, PPD
(Statens Seruminstitut Copenhagen) at final concentrations
of 0.05 and 0.01 mg/ml, Staphylococcus aureus vaccine at
12.5 and 50 mg/ml, tetanus toxoid at 0.75 and 0.075 U/ml,
cytomegalo virus and varicella 'complement fixing antigen'
and medium control, both diluted 200 times. The latter
antigens were obtained from the RIV, Bilthoven, The Netherlands.

RESULTS

Figures 2a and 2b give the PWM and Con A response of the
individual patients against time. Although the PHA LTT was
within the normal range before and after ATG treatment (data
not shown) this was not the case for the majority of the
patients when the responsiveness of their lymphocytes was
tested against PWM and Con A. It should be noted that the
lymphocytes of patients No. 2, 3 and 5 had before and after
ATG treatment a response within the normal range when tested
against PWM. Normal responses were obtained for patients
No. 2, 5 and 6 in the Con A mitogen LTT. Figure 2c summa-
rizes the results with the antigen LTT before and after
treatment with ATG (only the response to Varidase is shown).
Again in some of these patients (Nos. 3 and 6) the results
were generally speaking within normal limits before and
after ATG treatment. However, in the majority of the patients
the response against most antigens was abnormally low.
    One patient (No. 7) was studied in somewhat more detail.
Figure 1 shows the values of the peripheral blood elements
before and after ATG treatment. A sharp increase in the
numbers of all blood elements was noticed shortly after ATG
treatment and this made it unlikely that the amelioration

of the aplastic anemia was a coincidence.

Figure 3 details the mitogen, antigen-LTT, and the MLC and CML results obtained with the lymphocytes of patient No. 7 before and after treatment with ATG. The data in Figure 3 show the PHA LTT was within normal limits before and after ATG, but PWM, Con A, and antigen LTT's were low before ATG treatment and normalized after ATG treatment. The MLC test was low normal before and was slightly higher after ATG treatment. In contrast to these findings the CML was abnormally high before and normal, i.e. lower, after ATG treatment.

DISCUSSION

The results reported in this study document for the first time that the mitogen induced LTT and to a lesser extent the specific antigen induced LTT are abnormal in patients

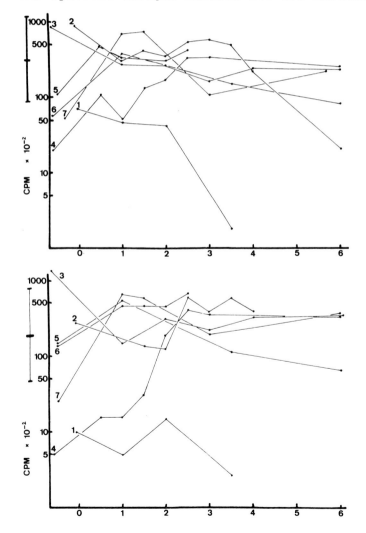

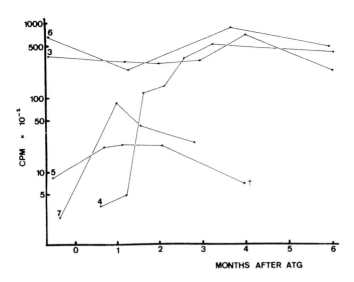

Fig. 2. Evolution of the hematological values after ATG. (a) Granulocytes mm^{-1}. (b) Reticulocytes in $^{0}/_{00}$. (c) Lymphocytes mm^{-1}.

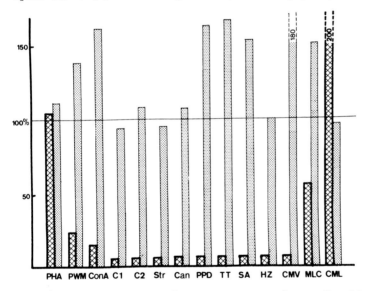

Fig. 3. Lymphocyte transformation test values of patient No. 7 and
cytotoxic capacity (CML) before ( ) and after ATG treatment ( ) in
percentage of the modal response of a pool of controls.

with aplastic anemia and can be normalized by ATG. These
findings are of importance at least in two aspects. In the
first place they lend further credibility to our working
hypothesis that ATG indeed can, if not cure, at least improve some patients suffering from aplastic anemia. Many
clinicians involved in the treatment of aplastic anemia
remain highly sceptical on this point. Other arguments which
led us to think that ATG is effective have been reviewed
before (1). In brief they include the fact that severely ill
patients improved after ATG treatment (see also Figure 1)
and that the bone marrow of aplastic anemia patients con-

36

tains T cells which interfere with the formation of CFU_C (2,3) and probably the differentiation of stem cells.

The question of how we should interpret these findings is of basic interest and whether they can help us interpret the pathogenesis of aplastic anemia. At least two mechanisms could be envisaged. The first is that the low LTT's are due to an increase of suppressor cells and the high CML test in patient No. 7 to a large number of cytolytic cells. Whether the suppressor and cytolytic cells belong to one lymphocyte population comparable to the Ly-2,3 cells of the mouse remains to be assessed. Speculating further one could wonder whether the effectiveness of the ATG might depend on its contents of the human analogue of anti Ly-2,3.

Whether the suppressor cells, the cytolytic cells, or both are responsible for the differentiation-block of the stem cells remains also to be assessed. Another possibility which we favor is that the primary pathogenic factor is the presence of a clone of cytolytic cells. These cells would have to be autoimmune in the sense that they will not react with the stem cells themselves (they can be shown to be present) but with for instance the committed stem cells of the patient. It could then be envisaged that the low LTT values obtained are due to the destruction of PWM, Con A or antigen induced blasts and not to suppression. This assumption is testable. It would be of interest also to ask whether the autologous PWM and Con A but not PHA induced blasts share antigens with the stem cells. The high CML is then also logical.

It is of interest that Goulmy found 3 instances of MHC restricted H-Y killing in 10 patients with aplastic anemia and none in 10 multitransfused patients with end-stage renal disease. This too could be interpreted as indicating that aplastic anemia is more prone to develop autoimmune MHC restricted cytolytic cells, which with relatively little priming can react with non-MHC targets.

As already pointed out in the introduction, many patients improve, but only a few are really cured from the aplastic anemia. If our assumptions are correct they indicate that immunosuppressive treatment with ATG is indicated but only partly effective. The studies presented here might help to define protocols to improve the treatment of aplastic anemia by immunosuppression.

ACKNOWLEDGEMENTS

We are indebted to A. Thompson and E. Goulmy for performing the LTT and CML tests respectively. We are grateful to J. van Nassau for her patience in typing the manuscripts.

REFERENCES

1. Speck, B., Gluckman, E., Haak, H.L. and Van Rood, J.J. (1977): Lancet, 2, 1145.
2. Haak, H.L., Goselink, H.M., Veenhof, W., Pellinkhof-Stadelmann, S.,

Kleivarda, J.K. and Te Velde, J. (1977): Scand. J. Haemat., 19, 159-171.

3. Ascensao, J., Kagan, W., Moorem, M., Pahea, R., Hansen, J. and Good, R. (1967): Lancet, 1, 669.

4. Goulmy, E., Termijtelen, A., Bradley, B.A. and Van Rood, J.J. (1976): Tissue Antigens, 8, 317-326.

5. Greaves, M., Janossy, G. and Doenhoff, M. (1974): J. exp. Med., 140, 1-18.

HUMAN-PLACENTA-CONDITIONED MEDIUM AS SOURCE OF COLONY-STIMULATING ACTIVITY FOR HUMAN GRANULOPOIETIC STEM CELL (CFU-C) CULTURES[*]

H.-P. Lohrmann

Department für Innere Medizin, Abteilung für Hämatologie, Ulm/Donau, Federal Republic of Germany

The in vitro culture of human granulopoietic stem cells (colony-forming units in culture, CFU-C) has provided a useful tool not only for the elucidation of the physiology and regulation of granulopoiesis, but also for the study of the pathogenesis of human hematological diseases. For this in vitro culture system, addition of a glycoprotein operationally defined as colony-stimulating factor (or in less pure preparation, colony-stimulating activity) is mandatory in order to observe colony formation. For human CFU-C cultures a double-layer culture system has been most widely used. In this system, a feeder layer containing normal human peripheral blood leukocytes provides the colony-stimulating activity necessary for the colony formation by target cells contained in the upper layer. Analytical studies have shown monocytes to be the primary source of CSA in this system [1,2], although segmented neutrophils are known to modify colony formation in this system [3].

For everybody working in the field, it has been a daily experience that colony stimulating using the double-layer agar culture system is variable, mainly depending on the composition and the source of the normal peripheral blood leukocytes contained in the feeder layer. This variability is of particular importance when one performs longitudinal studies of human CFU-C. We have encountered this problem studying the reaction of a normal human granulopoiesis to cytotoxic drug therapy. However, the same problem may be encountered in studies on the reconstitution of stem cells following bone marrow transplantation. We therefore would like to briefly review our experience with human-placenta-conditioned medium as a constant source of colony-stimulating activity for human CFU-C cultures.

METHODS

Human placentas were obtained without ligation of the umbilical cord, stored immediately at 4°C, and used within 6 hours after delivery. Preparations were performed in a laminar flow hood, on sterile plastic sheets. After removal

---

[*]A detailed report has appeared in <u>Blut</u>, 1978, 36, 81-88.

of the amniotic membrane, the placental tissue was cut into pieces of approximately 20 to 30 mm^3. These pieces were rinsed 3 times in RPMI 1640 containing penicillin, strepto-mycin and glutamin. Twenty-five pieces were placed into 250 ml plastic tissue culture bottles containing 40 ml of RPMI 1640, with the above-mentioned supplements plus 5% fetal calf serum. The loosely closed bottles were incubated flat at 37°C in a fully humidified atmosphere with 5% CO_2 in air. After 6 days, the medium was filtered through sterile gauze, pooled, centrifuged for 15 minutes at 3,000 x g and the supernatant filter-sterilized. This material was stored at -20°C until use and then used for cultures without further purification.

Bone marrow was aspirated under local anesthesia from the posterior iliac crest, anticoagulated with disodium-EDTA. Marrow particles were broken up by passage through needles of decreasing diameter. Red cells were sedimented at 37°C after admixture of 10% dextran. The supernatant con-taining the nucleated marrow cells was aspirated, washed twice and resuspended in supplemented McCoy's solution (4).

The double-layer system with human peripheral blood leukocytes in the feeder layer was used as previously de-scribed by our group (3). With human-placenta-conditioned medium (HPCM), 1-ml cultures were set up containing bone marrow cells in supplemented McCoy's solution, 15% fetal calf serum, 5% horse serum, and 0.3% agar. If not otherwise stated, 0.15-0.2 ml of HPCM were added per 1 ml culture. In the dose response studies, HPCM was serially diluted with supplemented McCoy's solution, and equal volumes of these dilutions were added per plate. To study the impact of seg-mented neutrophils (PMN) on HPCM-stimulated cultures, in-creasing numbers of PMN were added to single layer cultures of Ficoll-Isopaque separated bone marrow cells. These mar-row cells were devoid of mature granulocytes; thus, dif-ferences in colony growth could be ascribed to the granulo-cytes added.

Cultures were incubated for 10 days at 37° in sealed, humidified, CO_2-gassed glass containers (5). Colonies, de-fined as aggregates of more than 50 cells, were counted using a dissecting microscope.

RESULTS

The colony-stimulating capacity of 8 different batches of HPCM was compared to that of standard human leukocyte feeder layers. One batch did not support the formation of colonies, and two other batches did not stimulate to optimal levels. However, 5 batches stimulated the formation of colonies to the same levels as the leukocyte feeder layers did.

Dose-response curves showed a broad plateau, usually extending from 10 to 25% (with some batches, from 7.5 to 30%) of HPCM. At higher doses of HPCM (50%), there was neg-ligible colony growth; at lower doses, colony formation gradually declined.

Seven or 8 days of incubation were suboptimal for colony formation. Numbers and sizes of colonies were greatest on days 9 and 10.

Repeated studies showed a linear correlation between the number of marrow cells plated, and the number of colonies grown. This was true at optimal as well as at suboptimal concentrations of HPCM. The effect of varying concentrations of segmented neutrophils (PMN) within the culture plates on HPCM-stimulated colony growth from bone marrow target cells was studied. Up to 10^6 PMN per plate did not affect colony formation in this system.

DISCUSSION

The data presented indicate that crude, unseparated preparations of HPCM are a useful tool for routine assay of human CFU-C. 'Good' batches of HPCM are easily prepared, they have a broad plateau in the dose-response curve, there is a linear correlation between the number of marrow cells plated and the number of colonies grown, and the composition of bone marrow in terms of PMN content does not affect colony formation. Since HPCM can be stored frozen for extended periods, it appears to be preferable to the standard leukocyte feeder layer preparations so far used for stimulation of human CFU-C. Its advantages are: it is inexpensive to prepare, it is readily available in large quantities, it reduces the incidence of bacterial or fungal contaminations of cultures; and, most importantly, it offers a constant source of colony-stimulating activity for longitudinal studies.

REFERENCES

1. Chervenick, P.A. and Boggs, D.R. (1970): Human blood monocytes: stimulators of granulocyte and mononuclear colony formation in vitro. Science, 169, 691.
2. Golde, D.W. and Cline, M.J. (1972): Identification of the colony-stimulating cell in human peripheral blood. J. clin. Invest., 51, 2981.
3. Heit, W., Kern, P., Heimpel, H. and Kubanek, B. (1977): The role of granulocytes in colony stimulation by human white blood cells in agar cultures. Enhancement and inhibition of CSA. Scand. J. Haemat., 18, 105.
4. Pike, B.L. and Robinson, W.A. (1970): Human bone marrow colony growth in agar gel. J. cell. Physiol., 76, 77.
5. Firket, H. (1969): A very simple trick to produce controlled CO_2 concentrations in the gas phase overlying cell cultures. Experienta (Basel), 25, 671.

BONE MARROW TRANSPLANTATION IN APLASTIC ANEMIA:

A NEW CONDITIONING REGIMEN USING TOTAL IRRADIATION AND LUNG SHIELDING

E. Gluckman, A. Devergie, A. Bussel and J. Bernard

Centre Hayem, Hôpital Saint-Louis, Institut de Recherches sur les Maladies du Sang, Paris, France

SUMMARY

Treatment of severe aplastic anemia with allogeneic bone marrow graft. Report of 37 cases.

Thirty-seven patients with severe aplastic anemia received a bone marrow graft from an HLA identical sibling. Seventeen patients (46%) survived with a follow-up range from 53 days to 4 years. Twenty-seven patients were conditioned with cyclophosphamide (200 mg/kg) associated with or without antilymphocyte globulin and procarbazine. The main problem was marrow rejection which was found in 16 patients (59%). Among this rejection group, only 2 patients survived, one after auto-logous marrow reconstitution, the other after a second graft with another HLA identical sibling. Ten patients received cyclophosphamide 120 mg/kg associated with 800 rads total body irradiation with lung shielding (400 rads). No rejection was observed. The second problem was graft-versus-host-disease. This was observed in 8 cases. Four patients died; 2 had a complete recovery; 1 had chronic graft-versus-host-disease, and 1 is still under ALG. Eleven patients had an uneventful recovery after grafting. Two patients died of viral complications on day 68 and 130. This study shows the interest of a conditioning regimen including total body irradiation.

Bone marrow transplantation seems to be the best therapeutic approach for severe aplastic anemia. Severe aplastic anemia is defined by the results of blood counts when reticulocytes are less than $20,000/mm^3$, platelets less than $20,000/mm^3$ and granulocytes less than $500/mm^3$, with a depleted marrow. In the Hospital Saint-Louis Bone Marrow Transplant Unit, we have treated 37 consecutive aplastic patients which fulfilled this definition. The donor was an HLA identical sibling. During the study, 2 types of conditioning regimen were used.

From 1973-1977 patients received cyclophosphamide with or without procarbazine and ATG according to the Seattle group protocol. The number of rejections was found to be very high (59%). Therefore, since 1977 we have used a conditioning regimen according to the regimen used in conditioning leukemia patients, with slight modifications (5): viz., cyclophosphamide (120 mg/kg) associated with a 800-rads total body irradiation with a 400-rads lung shielding.

No rejection was observed. The overall results will be presented.

MATERIAL AND METHODS

Among 37 patients with severe aplastic anemia (SAA), 6 had post hepatitis AA, 1 chloramphenicol-induced AA, 2 Fanconi anemia, 28 idiopathic AA. The age range was from 3 to 29 years. They had all received androgens and 5 patients had had antilymphocyte globulin (ALG) treatment without success. All had received previous transfusions, but only 1 patient had a transfusion from a family member (mother). Twenty patients had anti-HLA antibodies and were refractory to random platelet transfusions. The donor was an HLA-A, B, C and D identical sibling. Seven patients were grafted against a major ABO incompatibility. Plasmapheresis was performed before and after grafting to remove agglutinins.

DECONTAMINATION AND TRANSFUSION

All the patients were isolated in reverse isolation rooms. Gut sterilization was achieved with oral non-absorbable antibiotics. They received a gluten-free sterile diet.
    Oral antifungal therapy was systematically given. Oral and skin decontamination was done with antiseptics. Blood support was given prophylactically to maintain hemoglobin levels above 8 g/100 ml and platelet levels above 20,000/mm^3. Granulocytes transfusions were given only if indicated by sepsis. All blood products had 2,500 rads irradiation.

CONDITIONING REGIMEN

Nine patients received procarbazine 12.5 mg/kg on days -10, -8 and -6 with ALG 7.5 mg/kg (Mérieux) on days -9, -7 and -5 and cyclophosphamide 50 mg/kg on days -6, -5, -4 and -3. Seventeen patients received on day -7 donor buffy coat and cyclophosphamide 50 mg/kg on days -6, -5, -4 and -3 (2). Ten patients received cyclophosphamide 60 mg/kg on days -4 and -3 and 1000-800 rads total body irradiation and 500 to 400 lung shielding with a dose rate ranging from 7 to 11.5 rads/min. Bone marrow aspiration and infusion followed the Seattle group protocol (4).
    After grafting, the patients received methotrexate 15 mg/sq.m on day 1, then 10 mg/sq.m on days 3, 6, 11. After this, the drug was administered weekly till day 100 to mitigate graft-versus-host-disease (GVHD).
    Chimerism was proved by genetic markers studies.

RESULTS (Table 1)

Two groups of patients were studied. The first group received cyclophosphamide with or without ALG and procarbazine and the second group cyclophosphamide and TBI.
    In the first group, 16 patients (59%) rejected their

TABLE 1. AA conditioning regimen and results

	Number of patients	Take	Reject	Severe GVHD	Number of patients alive
Chemotherapy	27	11	16	4	10[*]
		40.7%	59%	15%	37%
Cytoxan + TBI	10	10	0	4	7
		100%		40%	70%

[*]1 autologous reconstitution; 1 second BMT with a take.

graft. A second graft attempt was unsuccessful in 7 cases. Only 2 patients who rejected their graft survived; one after a second graft with another HLA-identical sibling, the other after autologous marrow reconstitution. The follow-up of anti-HLA antibodies was a good predictive test of rejection in pre-immunized patients (1). Eleven patients had a take, and severe GVHD was observed in 4 patients, which was treated with ALG.

Three patients died of GVHD and infectious complications. One patient is surviving without sequelae of GVHD. Seven patients had an uneventful recovery after grafting. They are fully chimeric with a follow-up ranging from 1-4 years.

The second group received TBI in addition to cyclophosphamide. The lung was shielded during the second half of irradiation to avoid interstitial pneumonitis, which is very frequent in leukemic patients who receive a 1,000 rads TBI. The irradiation was delivered by a linear accelerator (Neptune, Thomson)[*]. The first 2 patients received 1,000 rads with 500 rads to the lung. The next 3 patients received 800 rads with 400 rads to the lung with a dose rate of 7 rads/min. The last 5 patients received the same dose with a dose rate of 11 rads/min (Table 2).

The tolerance of irradiation was always good, except for nausea, chills, fever and a transient parotiditis during the second half of irradiation.

As seen in Table 3, no rejection was observed. Six patients had no or mild GVHD which was treated with corticosteroids. Four patients had severe GVHD which was treated with antilymphocyte globulin and placental globulins. Seven patients are still alive with a follow-up ranging from 53-383 days. Two patients have chronic hepatitis, 1 (patient 9) still has acute GVHD that is under treatment. The other surviving patients are doing well. Three patients died;

Pr DUTREIX - Institut Gustave Roussy, Villejuif.

TABLE 2. TBI with lung shielding

Patient	Abdomen dose (rads)	Lung dose (rads)	Dose rate (rad/min)	Source distance (m)	Length of irradiation (hr)	Actual dose rate (rad/min)
MEU	1087.5	549.5	7	5.6	7	2.58
JAC	939	569	7	5.6	5	3.13
JAM	796.5	514.5	7	5.6	4	3.3
BOI	765	489	7	5.6	4	3.2
BEN	815.5	449.5	7	5.6	4	3.4
MEG	756	402	11.5	4.20	3	4.5
VER	691	390	11.5	4.20	2 hr 30	4.5
FOL	761	365	11.5	4.20	3 hr 15	4.5
HEG	851	390	11.5	4.20	3	4.5
LUC	810	360	11.5	4.20	2 hr 30	4.5

one of severe GVHD, metabolic and infectious complications; one died of subacute necrotizing hepatitis, and one of CMV interstitial pneumonitis.

DISCUSSION

Our results show that 17 out of 37 patients (45.9%) are still alive after allogeneic transplantation for aplastic anemia. Two conditioning regimens have been studied consecutively. The first one follows the Seattle group protocol and 37% of the patients survived. The main cause of failure was rejection, which occurred in 59% of the cases. Rejection was not correlated in our series with the relative response index in mixed leukocyte culture, with the sex difference or with the number of marrow cells infused as it was described by Storb (3). It was certainly related to previous transfusions but 2 patients only had received less than 10 transfusions before grafting. The presence of anti-HLA antibodies before grafting had no predictive value. The follow-up of these antibodies was useful; their persistence was always associated with rejection.

These results suggest that the level of immunosuppression obtained with cyclophosphamide varies from one patient to another probably because of a different hepatic metabolism or urinary excretion of the drug.

As we are not able to predict graft rejection, we have preferred to use a conditioning regimen using total body irradiation which is known to obtain a marrow take in nearly all patients. Our protocol followed the regimen used by Thomas for conditioning patients with acute leukemia. It used cyclophosphamide 60 mg/kg x 2 and 1,000 rads total

TABLE 3. Conditioning with cyclophosphamide and 800 rads TBI

Patient	Age/Sex	Etiology	Anti-HLA antibodies	Number of cells/kg	Rejection	GVH	day	Survival days
MEU	16/F	Idiopathic	++++	3.5×10^8	0	III	9	+36 infectious and metabolic complications
JAC	22/M	Idiopathic	++++	3.3×10^8	0	III	7	>383 resolving chronic GVH
BEN	22/F	Idiopathic	++++	10×10^8	0	III	22	>242
BOI	29/F	Idiopathic	++++	2×10^8	0	I	14	†128 subacute necro-tizing hepatitis
JAM	19/M	Post-hepatitis	−	2.6×10^8	0	I	9	>194 chronic hepatitis
MEG	15/M	Idiopathic	−	3×10^8	0	II	120	>130
VER	22/F	Idiopathic	−	1.9×10^8	0	I	10	†63 CMV interstitial pneumonitis
FOL	13/M	Idiopathic	++++	3.5×10^8	0		0	>82
HEG	24/M	Post-hepatitis	++	1.6×10^8	0	III	28	>63 GVH still present
LUC	24/M	Idiopathic	−	1.8×10^8	0	II	50	>53

46

body irradiation.

The main problem in these patients is the high frequency of lethal interstitial pneumonitis. Its origin is multifactorial, related to opportunistic infections in immunosuppressed patients and also to the toxic effect of chemotherapy and irradiation on the lung. The role of irradiation in the genesis of this complication is controversial but we can just observe that it is more frequent in patients who have received this regimen. In an attempt to decrease this complication, we have purposely decreased the lung dose of irradiation because in aplastic anemia immunosuppression and not tumor killing is necessary.

For the same purpose, the total dose was decreased from 1,000 rads to 800 rads. Our results show that rejection was not observed in our patients.

Severe GVHD was observed in 4 cases and was the cause of death in 1 case. Persisting immune deficiency is still a problem and 2 patients died of viral infection despite mild GVHD. One of them died of CMV interstitial pneumonitis.

CONCLUSIONS

A conditioning regimen using TBI with lung shielding seems to solve the problems related to bone marrow graft rejection. Despite these encouraging results, it is too early to assess with certainty the superiority of this regimen over cyclophosphamide alone insofar as we do not yet have enough patients, nor a long-term follow-up. The main objective must be to find the minimum immunosuppressive regimen which gives 100% takes. This aim will be achieved if a good predictive test of rejection is available.

Another objective would be the prevention and treatment of GVHD and opportunistic infections related to persisting immune deficiency.

REFERENCES

1. Gluckman, E., Gluckman, J.C., Andersen, E., Devergie, A. and Dausset, J. (1979): Lymphocytotoxic antibodies and bone marrow grafts from HLA identical siblings - I HLA antibodies. Transplantation, in press.
2. Santos, G.W., Sensenbrenner, L.L., Burke, P.J., Mullins, G.M., Anderson, P.N., Tutshka, P.J., Braine, H.G., Davis, T.E., Humphrey, R.L., Abeloff, M.D., Bias, W.B., Borgaonkar, D.S. and Slavin, R.E. (1974): Allogeneic marrow grafts in man using cyclophosphamide. Transplant. Proc., 6, 345-348.
3. Storb, R., Prentice, R.L. et al. (1977): Marrow transplantation for treatment of aplastic anemia. An analysis of factors associated with graft rejection. New Engl. J. Med., 296, 61-66.
4. Thomas, E.D. and Storb, R. (1970): Technique for human marrow grafting. Blood, 36, 507-515.
5. Thomas, E.D., Storb, R., Clift, R.A., Fefer, A., Johnson, F.L., Neiman, P.E., Lerner, K.G., Glucksberg, H. and Buckner, C.D. (1975): Bone marrow transplantation. New Engl. J. Med., 292, 832-843 and 895-902.

MAJOR ABO-INCOMPATIBLE BONE MARROW TRANSPLANTATION

A. Bussel[1], C. Schenmetzler[1], E. Gluckman[2], A. Devergie[2]
and J. Reviron[1]

[1]Centre de Secteur de Transfusion, and [2]Unité de Recherche
sur les Maladies du Sang, Hôpital Saint-Louis, Paris,
France

SUMMARY

The role of the ABH system as potential target antigens of graft rejection was investigated in 10 recipients with antibodies directed against
the cells of their marrow donors. Plasma exchanges and antibody absorption in vivo were effective in permitting engraftment in 8/10 recipients. Complications and failure of these techniques are discussed.
These findings indicate that ABO-incompatible grafts should be considered in recipients with otherwise compatible donors.

Bone marrow transplantation has been used successfully in
various hematological disorders (1,2,11,12). Marrow donors
are usually selected from HLA-identical siblings. In order
to utilize donors who were otherwise ideally matched, we
have investigated the effectiveness of plasma exchange and
antibody absorption in vivo in preparing 10 recipients for
ABO-incompatible marrow transplants.

MATERIALS AND METHODS

Patients

The study included 10 patients, 2 with hematological malignancies and 8 with aplastic anemia. Detailed clinical information has already been published (5). All donor recipient pairs were HLA-A-, B- and D-compatible. Aplastic patients were conditioned for transplantation with cyclophosphamide or cyclophosphamide and total body irradiation. Patients with leukemia received various antileukemic agents
before conditioning with cyclophosphamide and total body
irradiation. After transplantation, patients received methotrexate to mitigate graft-versus-host disease.

Plasma exchange

Continuous flow plasma exchange was carried out with an IBM
blood cell separator operated at 100 x g. Flow into the
centrifuge was performed via teflon catheters or a surgic-
ally placed external arteriovenous fistula. Plasma (4/6
liters) was removed by exchange, and isometrically replaced

48

by donor-type fresh frozen plasma and 4% purified albumin using a ratio 1:1 by volume, respectively. Physiologic concentrations of calcium and potassium were added to all replacement fluids.

Antibody absorption in vivo

On completion of the last exchange, blood group substance A derived from porcine gastric mucosa (Benasil Corporation, Miami) or substance B from equine gastric mucosa (Benasil Corporation, Miami) was infused in patients Nr. 1, 2, 5 and 7. The required dose in vivo was estimated by an in vitro neutralization assay. All recipients were transfused with 1-2 units of donor-type packed red cells. In all instances, donor marrow was infused within 4 hours of completion of the plasma exchange. Post transplant patients Nr. 1 and 2 were transfused with blood products of donor ABO type. The other patients received red cells, granulocytes and platelets of their own ABO group; plasma was removed and replaced by plasma of donor ABO type.

ABO antibody titers

For IgM anti A and anti B titers, 2-fold serial dilutions of patient serum were reacted against a 2% suspension of donor ABO red cells for 2 hours at 4ºC. The tubes were read for microscopic agglutination. IgG anti A and anti B titers were determined as an indirect Coombs' test using an anti IgG globulin. All first serum samples were tested for immune antibody: anti A and anti B titers were determined as an indirect Coombs' test after serum absorption with blood group substance A or substance B and after heat denaturation.

Gene markers

Red blood cells obtained from peripheral blood were analyzed for ABO, Lewis, Rhesus, MNSs, Duffy, Kell, Kidd and P antigen systems. To determine the percentage of donor red cells in the transplant recipient, differential red cell agglutination in the ABO system was performed and results were expressed in comparison with a reference scale.

RESULTS

Engraftment and graft rejection

Engraftment was documented in 9/10 recipients (Table 1). Four recipients survived (Nrs. 7, 8, 9 and 10); patient 3 died from interstitial pneumonia on day 70. Three recipients died from graft-versus-host disease (Nrs. 1, 4 and 6).
    Evidence of hemolysis was documented in recipient Nr. 2 who received donor-type red cell transfusions after grafting in order to absorb in vivo a persistent antibody. In this

TABLE 1. Clinical data

Nr.	Age (yr)	Diagnosis	ABO Donor	Recipient	Engraftment	Survival (days)
1	18	C.M.L.	A_2	0	Yes	71
2	25	A.M.L.	A_1	0	Partial	32
3	22	A.A.	A_2	0	Yes	70
4	9	A.A.	A_1	0	Yes	45
5	15	A.A.	A_1	0	No	90
6	10	Fanconi A.	A_1	0	Yes	47
7	11	A.A.	B	0	Yes	>900
8	21	A.A.	A_1B	A_1	Yes	>290
9	29	A.A.	B	0	Yes	>120
10	29	A.A.	B	0	Yes	>110

Abbreviations: C.M.L., chronic myeloid leukemia. A.M.L., acute myelo-blastic leukemia. A.A., aplastic anemia. *Two bone marrow transplanta-tions with the same donor.

patient, evidence of engraftment was obtained but circulat-ing reticulocytes were never detected, although erythro-blasts were present in the marrow. The patient developed ascites and liver failure, which was the cause of death on day 32. The single recipient failing to engraft (Nr. 5) had received one platelet transfusion from an unrelated ABO-incompatible donor 3 weeks before transplantation. Subse-quent to the transplant, an anti A IgM titer of 1:16 and an anti IgG titer of 1:512 were demonstrated. On day 64, a second marrow graft was performed with the same donor. Anti A activity remained unmodified except for a short period when plasma exchanges were performed. Engraftment was again not observed (Fig. 1).

Removal of antibodies against donor ABO antigens

One to 3 plasma exchanges were performed in all recipients before absorption in vivo of ABO antibodies. Post transplant, 5/10 recipients needed 1-9 plasma exchanges to remove resid-ual ABO antibodies. The procedure was well tolerated without clinical evidence of hypocalcemia or bleeding.

An hypersensitivity reaction including chills, flushing and bronchospasm was observed in 2/4 recipients during in-fusion of blood group substance. One of these recipients had received previously antilymphocytic globulins of equine origin.

Hemolysis was not detected when donor-type erythrocytes

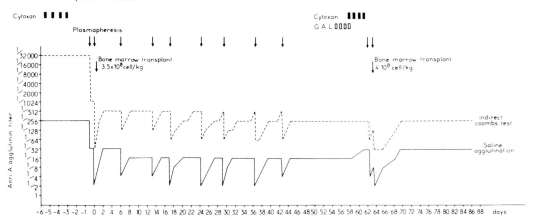

Fig. 1. IgM and IgG anti A antibody titers of patient Nr. 5.

or marrow donor were infused after completion of plasma exchanges. However, the direct Coombs' test was positive and was detected on incompatible donor-type red cells only using an anti IgG globulin. Anti A or anti B were regularly eluted from donor-type erythrocytes.

Anti A - anti B titers

Before conditioning for transplantation, recipients had IgM and IgG antibodies directed against ABO antigens present on the cells of their donors (Table 2). Recipient Nr. 5 had a high IgG titer with serological evidence of immune activity, which could be proved to be induced by an ABO-incompatible platelet transfusion. Before the platelet transfusion, IgM and IgG anti A titers were 1:64/1:256 respectively. Fifteen days later, anti A titers had increased to 1:256/1:32,000.

After plasma exchanges and absorption in vivo, low titers of IgM and IgG ABO antibodies were demonstrated in nearly all recipients before marrow infusion (Table 3).

During the first week after marrow infusion, demonstration of gradual increase of ABO antibody was obtained in 9/10 recipients (Table 4). In all cases, IgM and IgG titers were considerably lower than before transplantation. The outcome of persistent ABO antibodies was studied.

Antibody titers persisted unchanged in recipients Nr. 2 and 5 till their deaths on days 32 and 90 respectively. In recipient Nr. 2, an early attempt to absorb in vivo with donor-type erythrocytes transfusions was a failure and it induced hemolysis. In recipient Nr. 5, 2 marrow infusions were unsuccessful and plasma exchanges failed to modify synthesis of persistent antibody (see Fig. 1).

In 7 recipients, gradual antibody decrease was ob-

TABLE 2. Serological status of recipients before plasmapheresis

Recipient	ABO Donor	ABO Recipient	Saline titer	Coombs' titer	Coombs' titer After heating	Coombs' titer After absorption
1	A_2	O	1:32	1:32	1:2	1
2	A_1	O	1:256	1:512	1:16	1:32
3	A_2	O	1:32	1:32	1:2	1:2
4	A_1	O	1:64	1:256	0	1:8
5	A_1	O	1:256	1:32,000	1:1,024	1:1,024
6	A_1	O	1:32	1:64	1:4	0
7	B	O	1:64	1:1,024	1:4	1:32
8	A_1B	A_1	1:32	1:32	1:2	0
9	B	O	1:64	1:128	1:8	1:32
10	B	O	1:32	1:512	1:32	1:128

TABLE 3. Serological status of recipients before marrow infusion

Number	Antibody titer after plasma exchange IgM	Antibody titer after plasma exchange IgG	Antibody titer before marrow infusion IgM	Antibody titer before marrow infusion IgG
1	0	0	0	0
2	1:4	1:4	1	1
3	1:2	1	1	0
4	1:8	1:8	0	1:2
5	1:4	1:256	1:2	1:32
6	1	1:4	0	0
7	1:16	1:32	1:2	1:2
8	1	1	0	0
9	1:8	1:16	1:4	1:4
10	1	1:32	0	1:4

served 4 weeks after transplantation. In 3 of them, plasma exchanges were performed systematically. Thereafter, progressive decrease of antibodies was observed when circulating donor erythrocytes were detected. In 4 recipients, plasma exchanges were not performed and decrease of antibodies was spontaneously observed, although the IgG ABO antibody titer of recipient Nr. 3 was as high as 1:16. Absorption in vivo

TABLE 4. Residual ABO antibody titers

Recipient	ABO antibody titer		Number of plasma exchanges post grafting	Erythroid reconstitution
	IGM	IgG		
1	0	0	0	Yes
2	1:32	1:32	1	No
3	1:16	1:16	0	Yes
4	1:16	1:16	2	Yes
5	1:16	1:512	9	No
6	1:16	1:16	0	Yes
7	1:32	1:128	1	Yes
8	1:2	1:2	0	Yes
9	1:32	1:32	1	Yes
10	1:8	1:16	0	Yes

TABLE 5. Serological data of recipients with gradual antibody decrease

Number	3	4	6	7	8	9	10
Positive elution days	25→36	Negative	26→33	38→44	29→33	Negative	Negative
ABO antibody disappearance days	50	38	x	50	50	41	36

x = Persisting on day 47 when recipient died.

of antibodies was demonstrated by elution in some patients (Table 5).

Erythroid reconstitution

In order to study erythroid reconstitution, ABO markers were used in 6 recipients who did not receive donor-type red cells post transplantation and who survived long enough (Table 6).
    In all cases, circulating donor cells appeared almost at the same period, between the 4th and the 5th week post transplantation. In 4 recipients, complete reconstitution was observed on days 107, 120, 140 and 142.

TABLE 6. Erythroid reconstitution

Recipient	Donor red cells appearance (days post grafting)	Circulating donor red cells	
		%	Days post grafting
3	25	40	70[+]
4	28	25	45[+]
6	26	10	47[+]
7	31	100	107
8	23	100	142
9	32	100	120
10	25	100	140

[+]Day of death.

DISCUSSION

Among the techniques used to remove ABO antibodies, plasma exchange was the best tolerated. Before marrow infusion, 1-3 exchanges have been effective in permitting absorption in vivo of residual ABO antibodies without evidence of hemolysis. Post transplantation, erythroid reconstitutions could be obtained without any more plasma exchange in recipients with IgG ABO antibody titers $\leqslant 1/16$.

In contrast, some complications were observed after absorption in vivo. Infusion of blood group substance was associated with hypersensitivity reactions in 2 recipients. Such manifestations have been reported after repeated intravenous administration of blood group substance in volunteers (8). Whether immune complex disease or anaphylactic reactions were involved remains unknown.

Post transplantation donor-type erythrocyte transfusion resulted in a severe episode of hemolysis in a recipient who died from liver failure shortly afterwards. Gale (4) observed a patient who developed liver failure under similar circumstances. These observations suggested that an attempt to absorb in vivo with red cell transfusions post transplantation might not be safe in recipients with circulating incompatible ABO antibodies.

Increase of anti-donor ABO antibodies following transplantation was observed in all recipients but one. This finding could be explained by antibody diffusion from the extravascular space after plasma exchanges and/or by persisting recipient B lymphocyte function. In our experience, this latter explanation appeared likely. A similar observation has been made by Thomas (12) and Gale (4).

Despite residual antibodies relevant to A or B antigens on donor cells, occurrence and rate of erythroid reconstitution were not different from that of ABO-identical grafts in 7/9 recipients.

54

Occurrence of reconstitution was always associated with progressive decrease of anti-donor ABO antibody. This finding and evidence of circulating donor erythrocytes transiently coated with recipient antibody suggested that spontaneous absorption in vivo occurred. Whether the failure to detect thereafter circulating antibody is related to persistent absorption in vivo or to specific tolerance remains uncertain.

Demonstration of residual antibodies was associated with failure of erythroid reconstitution in recipient Nr. 2 and with marrow rejection in recipient Nr. 5. Whether these failures were related or not to more severe ABO-incompatibility between donors and recipients is questionable (10).

Indeed, it has to be pointed out that these recipients had been immunized against A antigens and had high anti A IgG titer post transplantation. Hemolysins anti A were found in patient Nr. 5 but not in patient Nr. 2. These 2 patients had peculiar antibodies of group O people (9) and their donors were of A_1 type. A_1 red cells are different from A_2 red cells in regard to the number of A antigenic sites (3) and the presence of A_p receptors (13).

It has been reported that the ABO group system does not play a significant role as a transplantation antigen in marrow grafting (4). However, only 13 bone marrow transplantations have been performed in hematological disorders using major ABO non-identical siblings (4,6,7,10,12). Three of them failed to engraft. These data do not allow conclusions to be drawn concerning possible immunological differences between donor-recipient pairs in regard to the degree of ABO-incompatibility.

Our transplant experience indicates that the ABO system is not a clinically significant barrier to complete engraftment in most cases. However, continued investigations will possibly specify some limitations in use of ABO-incompatible grafts.

REFERENCES

1. Camitta, B.M., Thomas, E.D., Santo, S.G., Gordon-Smith, E.C., Gale, R.P., Rappeport, J.M. and Storb, R. (1976): Severe aplastic anemia: A prospective study of the effect of early marrow transplantation in severe aplastic anemia. Lancet, 2, 921.
2. Cline, M.J., Gale, R.P., Stiehm, E.R., Opelz, G., Young, L.S. and Feig, S.A. (1975): Bone marrow transplantation in man. Ann. intern. Med., 83, 691.
3. Economidou, J., Hugues-Jones, N.C. and Gardner, B. (1967): Quantitative measurement concerning A and B sites. Vox Sang. (Basel), 12, 321.
4. Gale, R.P., Feig, S., Ho, W., Falk, P., Ripee, C. and Sparkes, R. (1977): ABO blood group system and bone marrow transplantation. Blood, 50, 185.
5. Gluckman, E., Devergie, A., Marty, M., Bussel, A., Rottembourg, J., Dausset, J. and Bernard, J. (1978): Allogeneic bone marrow transplantation in aplastic anemia. Report of 25 cases. Transplant.

Proc., 10, 141.

6. Graw Jr, R.G., Yankee, R.A., Leventhal, B.G., Rogentine, G.N., Herziq, G.P., Halterman, R.H., Merritt, C.B., Carolla, R.L., Alvegard, T.A., Bull, J.M., McGinniss, M.H., Krueger, G.R.D., Gullion, D.S., Lippman, M.H., Bleyer, W.A., Berard, C.W., Whang-Peng, J., Traprani, R.S., Terasati, P.I., Steinberg, A.S., Gralnick, H.R. and Henderson, E.S. (1972): Bone marrow transplantation in acute leukemia employing cyclophosphamide. Exp. Hemat., 22, 118.

7. Marmont, A.M., Damasio, E.E., Giordano, D., Rossi, E., Reali, G., Gay, A., Dagna-Bricarelli, F., Brema, F., Carella, A.M. and Santini, G. (1977): A to O bone marrow transplantation in severe aplastic anaemia. Dynamics of blood group conversion and demonstration of early dyserythroporesis in the engrafted marrow. Brit. J. Haemat., 36, 511.

8. McNeil, C., Covington, F.H. and O'Donnell, M.M. (1950): The effect of intravenous administration of large doses of A and B substances. Amer. J. clin. Path., 20, 349.

9. Race, R.R. and Sanger, R. (1975): Cross Reacting Anti A and Anti B in Group O Serum, p. 48. Blackwell Ed., Oxford.

10. Storb, R., Prentice, R.L. and Thomas, E. (1977): Marrow transplantation for treatment of aplastic anemia. An analysis of factors associated with rejection. New Engl. J. Med., 296, 61.

11. Storb, R., Thomas, E.D., Buckner, C.D., Clift, R.A., Johnson, F.L., Fefer, A., Glucksberg, H., Giblett, E.R., Lerner, K.G. and Neiman, P. (1974): Allogenic marrow grafting for treatment of aplastic anemia. Blood, 43, 157.

12. Thomas, E.D., Buckner, C.D., Banaji, M., Clift, R.A., Fefer, A., Flournoy, N., Goodell, B.W., Hickman, R.O., Lerner, K.G., Neiman, P.E., Sale, G.E., Sanders, J.E., Singer, J., Stevens, M., Storb, R. and Weiden, P.L. (1977): One hundred patients with acute leukemia treated by chemotherapy, total body irradiation and allogeneic marrow transplantation. Blood, 49, 511.

13. Winstanley, D.P., Konugres, A. and Coombs, R.R.A. (1957): Studies on human anti-A antigen and the specificity of the hemolysin in anti-A sera. Brit. J. Haemat., 3, 341.

56

THE DETECTION OF NON-HLA ANTIBODIES AND THEIR SIGNIFICANCE IN BONE MARROW GRAFT REJECTION

F.H.J. Claas[1], J.J. van Rood[1], R.P. Warren[2], R. Storb[2], P.L. Weiden[2] and P.J. Su[2]

[1]Department of Immunohaematology, University Hospital, Leiden, The Netherlands, and [2]Fred Hutchinson Cancer Research Center, Seattle, Washington, U.S.A.

Although bone marrow transplantation of an HLA-identical sibling is an effective form of therapy for patients with severe aplastic anemia, in about 30% of the cases the therapy fails, because of rejection of the bone marrow. The fact that grafts are still rejected with HLA identity and negative mixed lymphocyte reaction strongly suggests the presence of transplantation antigens, other than those of the HLA system. It is likely that graft rejection is due to sensitization of the recipient by blood transfusions to those non-HLA antigens before grafting (6). Attempts to identify presensitization of potential graft recipients to non-HLA antigens have generally failed, when the standard complement depending cytotoxicity test was used (8). Direct or antibody dependent cell mediated cytotoxicity against non-HLA antigens has however been reported to yield positive results (3,9). Warren et al. (7) have reported that a positive antibody dependent cell mediated cytotoxicity (ADCC) test of the serum of aplastic anemia patients against their respective HLA identical sibling donors correlated significantly with bone marrow rejection. Although the ADCC test is sensitive, it is also difficult to standardize, it is time consuming and it requires large amounts of cells and serum. For that reason we studied pretransplant sera of aplastic anemia patients for non-HLA antibodies in three different serological techniques.

MATERIALS AND METHODS

Sera from 16 aplastic anemia patients (from the Seattle group) were tested.

ADCC test

The antibody dependent cell mediated cytotoxicity (ADCC) tests were performed in Seattle as previously described (7). The ADCC tests were carried out with serum of the patients against the lymphocytes of their respective donors.

Serological techniques

For the serum of each aplastic anemia patient a panel of

2-8 unrelated individuals, HLA-A, -B, and -C identical to the serum donor (patient), was selected. The serum of each patient was tested against his panel in the following serological techniques: the EDTA micro-agglutination test (Van Rood et al. (4)), the Indirect ImmunoFluorescence test (Van Leeuwen et al. (2), modified by Décary et al. (1)), and the Two Colour Fluorescence test, a complement dependent cytotoxicity assay in which one can distinguish B-cells, T-cells and monocytes (Van Rood et al. (5)). These serological tests were considered to be positive if the serum of the patient showed a positive reaction with one or more individuals of the panel. As a control for the presence of anti-HLA antibodies, the sera were tested against a panel of 5 unrelated individuals, HLA non-identical to the serum donors.

RESULTS

The ADCC test with the serum of the patients against the lymphocytes of their respective HLA-identical sibling donors was positive in 8 of the 16 combinations tested.

The serum of the same 16 patients was tested in the three serological techniques against a panel of unrelated individuals, HLA-A, -B, and -C identical to the serum donor, i.e. the patient who received the bone marrow transplant. The EDTA micro-agglutination test was negative in all cases. In the Two Colour Fluorescence (TCF) test and the indirect immunofluorescence test, some sera showed positive reactions with all or part of the panel lymphocytes.

In Table 1 the reaction pattern of the serum of a patient against his HLA-A, -B, and -C identical panel is shown. In this case the monocytes of all panel donors were positive in the TCF test. In the indirect immunofluorescence test, also the B-cells of 2 of the 5 donors were positive. It is remarkable that only the B-cells of the female donors

TABLE 1. Serum of patient O.D.

Cell donor	Sex	DRw	TCF			IF		
			B	M	T	B	M	T
J.P.	F	3	−	+	−	+	+	−
H.C.	M	3	−	+	−	−	+	−
M.J.	M	2+3	−	+	−	−	+	−
E.B.	F	3	−	+	−	+	+	−
M.S.	M	2+3	−	+	−	−	+	−

were positive in the indirect immunofluorescence test, while the B-cells of the males were negative. This effect is not caused by difference in the known DRw antigens.

Generally not all members of the panel were positive with a serum, in some cases only 1 or 2 individuals were positive. Some sera were negative in the TCF test and positive in the indirect immunofluorescence test, never the other way around. If one or more members of a panel were positive with a certain serum, that serum was considered to be positive. In Table 2, the reactions of the sera as tested by TCF and indirect immunofluorescence against the HLA-A, -B, and -C identical panel were compared with the reactions in the ADCC test against the HLA-identical sibling donors.

TABLE 2. Sera tested against a panel of donors HLA-A, -B, -C identical with the serum donor

		TCF and/or IF	
		+	-
ADCC test	+	8	0
	-	2	6

There is a significant correlation between the ADCC test against the bone marrow donor and the serological reactions against the panel of HLA-A, -B, and -C identical individuals (p = 0.0035). All sera which were positive in the ADCC test, were also positive in the TCF test and/or in the indirect immunofluorescence test and 6 of the 8 ADCC negative sera were also negative in the serological tests. In two cases the serological tests were positive, while ADCC was negative.

As a control, the sera were also tested against a panel of individuals, HLA non-identical to the serum donor. Table 3 shows that there is no significant difference between the ADCC positive and the ADCC negative group. The sera of both groups contain anti-HLA antibodies.

TABLE 3. Sera tested against a panel of donors HLA-A, -B, -C non-identical with the serum donor

		TCF and/or IF	
		+	-
ADCC test	+	8	0
	-	7	1

Next the significance in bone marrow rejection of the detected anti-non-HLA antibodies was studied. Of the 8 patients who were positive in ADCC against their HLA-identical bone marrow donor, 3 rejected their bone marrow graft, while none of the 8 ADCC negative combinations showed rejection. However, this difference in rejection pattern between the ADCC positive and the ADCC negative group was not significant (p = 0.1).

Five out of the 16 sera tested showed positive reactions against the monocytes of some or all members of their HLA-A, -B, and -C identical panel in the Two Colour Fluorescence test. Table 4 shows that there is a significant correlation between a positive reaction of the serum against the monocytes of some or all members of the panel and rejection of the bone marrow graft (p = 0.03). Of the 5 patients

TABLE 4. Correlation between the presence of anti-monocyte antibodies in the serum and rejection of the bone marrow graft

		rejection	
		+	-
anti-monocyte antibodies (TCF)	+	3	2
	-	0	11

whose sera contained anti-monocyte antibodies against the panel, 3 rejected their bone marrow graft. The 3 patients with anti-monocyte antibodies, who rejected their graft, were positive in ADCC against their respective HLA identical sibling donors, while the 2 patients with anti-monocyte antibodies, who did not reject their graft, were negative in ADCC.

It is concluded that the sera which were positive in ADCC against the bone marrow donors and which contained anti-monocyte sera against the HLA-A, -B, and -C identical panel, had the best correlation (p = 0.0018) with rejection of the bone marrow graft.

DISCUSSION

Warren et al. (7) have reported that a positive ADCC test of the serum of aplastic anemia patients against their respective HLA-identical sibling donors correlates significantly with bone marrow rejection. This correlation was found in patients pretreated with cyclophosphamide. In the present study, the patients were pretreated with total body irradiation and cyclophosphamide. After this treatment no significant correlation was found between a positive ADCC against the bone marrow donor and rejection of the bone

TABLE 5. Sera with anti-monocyte antibodies in the TCF test and positive in ADCC show a significant correlation (p = 0.0018) with rejection of the bone marrow graft

		rejection	
		+	-
antibodies against monocytes and ADCC test	+	3	0
	-	0	13

marrow graft. The serum of the aplastic anemia patients was tested in three different serological techniques against a panel of unrelated individuals, HLA-A, -B, and -C identical with the serum donor (patient). A significant correlation was found between the reactions of the serum in ADCC against the bone marrow donor and the serological reactions against the panel. There was a significant correlation between rejection of the bone marrow graft and the presence of anti-monocyte antibodies, as detected in the Two Colour Fluorescence test. However, sera which were positive in ADCC against the HLA-identical sibling donor and which contained anti-monocyte antibodies against the HLA-identical panel, showed the best correlation with rejection of the bone marrow graft. These data indicate that the sera of aplastic anemia patients contained antibodies, which were not anti-HLA-A, -B, and -C or DRw and which were as well recognized by the serological methods used here as by the ADCC test. Family studies have to point out if the determinants recognized on monocytes are coded for by a locus of the HLA-complex or another locus outside HLA.

Our experiments show that the potential clinical significance of non-HLA antibodies, detected by the ADCC test, in combination with the presence of anti-monocyte antibodies in the TCF test, to grafted patients is considerable.

REFERENCES

1. Décary, F., Vermeulen, A. and Engelfriet, C.P. (1975): A look at HL-A antisera in the indirect immunofluorescence technique (IIFT). In: Histocompatibility Testing 1975, pp. 380-390. Munksgaard, Copenhagen.
2. Van Leeuwen, A., Schuit, H.R.E. and Van Rood, J.J. (1973): Typing for MLC (TD). The selection of non-stimulator cells by MLC inhibition tests using SD-identical stimulator cells (MISIS) and fluorescence antibody studies. Transplant. Proc., 5, 1539-1542.
3. Mawas, C., Christen, Y., Legrand, L., Sasportes, M. and Dausset, J. (1974): Cellular and humoral response against determinants other than the classical HL-A specificities. Transplantation, 18, 256-266.
4. Van Rood, J.J., Van Leeuwen, A. and Zweerus, R. (1970): The 4a and

4b antigens. Do they or don't they? In: Histocompatibility Testing 1970, pp. 93-103. Munksgaard, Copenhagen.

5. Van Rood, J.J., Van Leeuwen, A. and Ploem, J.S. (1976): Simultaneous detection of two cell populations by two colour fluorescence and application to the recognition of B-cell determinants. Nature (Lond.), 262, 795-797.

6. Storb, R., Rudolph, R.H., Graham, T.C. and Thomas, E.D. (1971): The influence of transfusions from unrelated donors upon marrow grafts between histocompatible canine siblings. J. Immunol., 107, 409-413.

7. Warren, R.P., Storb, R., Weiden, P.L., Mickelson, E.M. and Thomas, E.D. (1976): Direct and antibody dependent cell mediated cytotoxicity against HLA-identical sibling lymphocytes. Transplantation, 22, 631-635.

8. Wunderlich, J.R., Rogentine, C.N. and Yankee, R.A. (1972): Rapid in vitro detection of cellular immunity in man against freshly explanted allogeneic cells. Transplantation, 13, 31-37.

9. Yust, I., Wunderlich, J., Mann, D.L., Rogentine, C.N., Leventhal, B., Yankee, R. and Graw, R. (1974): Human lymphocyte dependent antibody mediated cytotoxicity and direct lymphocyte cytotoxicity against non-HLA antigens. Nature (Lond.), 249, 263-265.

II. Acute leukaemia

CURRENT STATUS AND PERSPECTIVES IN THE TREATMENT OF ACUTE
LEUKEMIA BY BONE MARROW TRANSPLANTATION[x]

B. Speck, W. Weber, P. Cornu, C. Nissen, P. Groff and
J. Sartorius[o]

Section of Hematology, Department of Internal Medicine,
Kantonsspital Basel and Kinderspital Basel[o], Switzerland

SUMMARY

Allogeneic bone marrow transplantation performed after chemotherapy
and total body irradiation is a treatment modality for acute leukemia
with the potential of cure for some patients. The major fatal complications have been interstitial pneumonia, graft-versus-host disease,
recurrence of leukemia and infection.
    The Basel experience with 13 end-stage leukemic patients showed
that the addition of polychemotherapy to the standard conditioning
programs of high-dose cyclophosphamide and total body irradiation has
probably increased the incidence of interstitial pneumonia without
eliminating the risk of developing recurrent leukemia. Based on our
experience and data that became available very recently we suggest that
bone marrow transplantation should be performed early in the course of
acute leukemia at a stage with a small tumor load and with a minimum
of drug induced organ damage.

In recent years progress in conventional chemo- and immunotherapy of acute leukemias has been disappointing. This has
prompted a resurgence of interest in clinical bone marrow
transplantation (BMT). The basic immunobiology of isogeneic
and allogeneic BMT in man has been documented, and recently
large series of patients with acute leukemia treated by this
modality became available (1-3). Most centers have been
using 1000 rad total body irradiation (TBI) for conditioning
patients. TBI provides sufficient immunosuppression to allow
for a take of allogeneic marrow. In addition it has good
antileukemic properties which seem to be particularly relevant for sites such as the central nervous system and the
gonads. If TBI was used as sole conditioning regimen for
acute leukemia, a high relapse rate was observed (2). In
two instances recurrent leukemia was documented in donor
cells (4). This prompted the use of high dose cyclophosphamide (Cy 2x60 mg/kg) prior to TBI. With this regimen no more
relapses in donor cells were seen, but recurrence of the
original leukemia remained a serious problem (2).

[x]Supported by the Swiss Cancer League Grants FOR 080.AK.75 and FOR
   101.AK.77 (2) and the Swiss Science Foundation Grant 3.3320.74.

65

BASEL EXPERIENCE

In a series of 13 consecutive patients with refractory acute
leukemia we tried to reduce the risk of leukemic relapse by
adding a 5-day course of polychemotherapy to the standard
Cy + TBI program. It consisted of vincristine (VCR), 1-(2-
chloroethyl)-3-cyclohexyl-1-nitrosourea (CCNU), busulfan,
cytosine arabinoside (Ara-C), 4'-demethyl(9-(4,6-O-2-theny-
lidene)-β-D-glucopyranoside)epipodophyllotoxin (VM-26) and
prednisone. TBI was given from a linear accelerator at a
dose rate of 7.5 rad/min. The first 11 patients were given
1000 rad midline tissue dose and the last two 500 rad.
    Seven patients had acute myelogenous leukemia (AML), 5
acute lymphoblastic leukemia (ALL) and one acute undifferentiated leukemia (Table 1). The median age was 18 years. Nine
patients were grafted in complete relapse. The patient with
acute undifferentiated leukemia (AUL) never reached a remission. Four patients were transplanted in partial relapse.
All patients were decontaminated with non-absorbable antibiotics and mycostatics and were given skin cleansing. In

TABLE 1. Details on 13 patients with end-stage acute leukemia who underwent allogeneic bone marrow transplantation after polychemotherapy,
high-dose cyclophosphamide and total body irradiation

Age (median, range)		18 (8 - 34)
Type of leukemia	AML	7
	ALL	5
	AUL	1
Sex male / female		8/5
Status at transplantation		
	Relapse	9
	Part. remission	4
Duration of chemotherapy prior to transplantation (months)		
	(median, range)	14 (6 - 52)

most instances gentamycin, vancomycin and mycostatin were
used. Eleven patients were nursed in ultrasterile protective
isolation units, 2 in single rooms with all possible aseptic
precautions.
    As donors we used exclusively HLA identical siblings
who were non-reactive in the mixed lymphocyte culture (Table
2). The patient with AUL had blood group AB, the donor A.
Marrow was aspirated from the pelvis in general anesthesia,
pooled, filtered and given intravenously. The median cell
number given was 2.9 x 10^8/kg (1.8-4.0 x 10^8/kg).

TABLE 2. Details on 13 sibling bone marrow donors

HLA identical		
MLC non reactive		
ABO identical	10	
major barrier	2	1 A → O
		1 AB → B
minor	1	1 A → AB
Sex identical	3	(2 m → m, 1 f → f)
non identical	10	(6 f → m, 4 m → f)
Marrow dose	2.9×10^{8}	(1.8 - 4.0)

In 12 instances prompt hemopoietic engraftment could be documented by repopulation of the marrow, rising blood counts and genetic markers. One patient died too early for evaluation (day 10). The one with AUL became a long-term survivor. He never showed any evidence of graft-versus-host disease (GVHD). At present he is a complete hemopoietic chimera without any detectable signs of leukemia at over 3 years post grafting and he is leading a normal life. His only minor problem is cataracts.

Recurrent leukemia occurred in 2 cases (Fig. 1). In one it was the cause of death at day 200, in the other it was found at autopsy in a patient who died from GVHD on day 56. GVHD occurred in 6 patients; 4 died of it between days 40 and 70 (median: 48 days) despite treatment with corticosteroids and antilymphocyte globulin (ATG). Cardiac toxicity

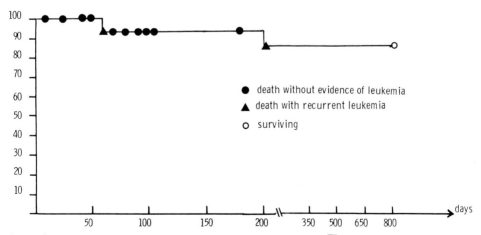

Fig. 1. Recurrences of acute leukemia in 13 patients who had polychemotherapy, total body irradiation and bone marrow transplantation.

caused the death of 1 patient.

Six patients died from interstitial pneumonia (IP) 20 to 180 days (median: 69 days) after transplantation. Twice it occurred during severe GvHD, 4 times GvHD was absent. In 5 instances the IP was classified as idiopathic, only once cultural and histological evidence for the presence of cytomegalovirus (CMV) could be found. IP usually started with a non-productive cough without physical findings and a fuzzy infiltrate on the chest X-ray. It was rapidly progressive in all cases and led to death from anoxia within 1 to 2 weeks. Treatment with adenine arabinoside (Ara-A), interferon, pentamidine, trimethoprimsulfamethoxazol (Bactrim), broad spectrum antibiotics, mycostatics and assisted ventilation on respirators with positive end expiratory pressure did not alter the relentless course of the disease. At autopsy pulmonary vessels showed severe alterations. In the small arteries mediolysis was found and a large amount of venules were obstructed by intimal edema. CMV was isolated in only one case. In 5 patients no pathogens and no lesions suggestive of infection were found.

INTERNATIONAL EXPERIENCE

In 1976 R.P. Gale reported the experience of a cooperative group for BMT in AL (5). In 217 allogeneic marrow grafts there was a 70% mortality in the first 6 months which was primarily due to GvHD and IP. Later deaths were mainly on account of leukemic relapse. The results were not significantly different for ALL and AML. In 100 grafts recently reported by the Seattle group 13% of patients survived 2 years and have a real chance to be cured, because leukemic relapse becomes extremely rare after this time span (2). The U.C.L.A. group reported that 5 out of 33 patients survived more than 1 to more than 2½ years in hematological remission after allogeneic BMT (1).

Grafts between identical twins are considerably better. In the Seattle series 6 out of 16 patients with syngeneic grafts for acute leukemia are in complete remission for more than 4 to more than 6½ years after transplantation (37.5%) (6).

In their recent analysis of 100 marrow grafts for AL the Seattle group proposed 4 grades of candidates for BMT based on the assessment of the clinical condition (Table 3) (2). No patients of grade 0 were referred for BMT. Of the grade 1 and 2 patients approximately 25% have a chance of becoming long-term survivors while after grade 3 and 4 the chance is only in the range of 5%. In a very recent study the duration of chemotherapy prior to transplantation was found to be the most important factor for the prognosis of the graft (7). Patients with over 8 months chemotherapy did significantly poorer than those with less.

TABLE 3. Assessment of the clinical condition at the time of transplantation in patients with acute leukemia (Thomas, E.D. et al. 1977, Ref. 2)

Grade	Parameters
0	CR, no transf.
1	CR or PR, transf. good clin. cond.
2	Relapse, no fever fair clin. cond.
3	Relapse, no fever, requiring platelet transf. and/or febrile, poor clin. cond.
4	Advanced relapse, and/or refractory to random platelets, and/or febrile on broad spectrum antibiotics, very poor clin. cond.

DISCUSSION AND CONCLUSIONS

To the best of our knowledge all patients who had chemotherapy alone for conditioning and who have an adequately long follow-up, died from recurrent leukemia. This was our main reason for including TBI in the conditioning program.

Adding polychemotherapy to the standard Cy + TBI program probably increased the incidence of IP which in our series always took a fatal course. The U.C.L.A. group has abandoned SCARI, a combined chemotherapy regimen used before Cy and TBI because of its serious toxicity with a high incidence of fatal infections. Our aggressive strategy has not eliminated the risk of developing recurrent leukemia and it is impossible to say if it has decreased it, because the majority of our patients have not been at risk for relapse for sufficiently long periods.

GVHD occurred in 50% of the patients despite perfect histocompatibility matching and prophylactic methotrexate (MTX). This indicates that antigens outside of the MHC are responsible for this complication and that MTX is certainly not an optimal prophylactic agent. ATG and steroids have not improved the prognosis of severe GvHD significantly either.

Studies on clinical BMT as a new mode of treatment of AL have been mainly pioneered by the Seattle group. They have shown that long-term survival without maintenance chemotherapy with a real chance of cure is possible. Chances of surviving BMT and of being cured seem to be considerably better if they are performed early in the disease; this is when the patient has not yet been exposed to large amounts of cytostatic agents and when his leukemic cell burden is relatively small (2,3). Under such optimal circumstances long-term survival can be expected to exceed 50% (3). Our

69

long-term survivor had the shortest chemotherapy in our
series. The fact that the duration of therapy prior to
transplantation is of crucial importance for the outcome of
the graft has been clearly documented in a recent cooperative international study (7).

At the moment marrow grafts for AL can only be performed in patients with HLA identical siblings. In our experience at the most 20% of the patients are in the situation of having such a donor. Furthermore it has to be borne
in mind that e.g. in the Seattle series the oldest long-term
survivor is 36 years old. Progress in histocompatibility
typing may make the use of histocompatible unrelated donors
feasible for a much larger proportion of patients within the
next few years.

We think that allogeneic BMT cannot be considered as a
purely experimental procedure in the treatment of AL anymore.
In order to definitely establish its place it should be compared with the best known conventional chemo- and chemoim-
munotherapy programs in a randomized fashion.

Of course much work has still to be done for the prevention and treatment of early fatal complications such as
IP and GvHD and also for the prevention of late problems
such as leukemic relapse and for improving the slow immunological reconstitution after BMT which takes at least one
year. BMT is an extremely difficult procedure. For the time
being a few highly specialized centers should continue this
endeavor until its real value is firmly established.

REFERENCES

1. Gale, R.P. et al. (1977): Bone marrow transplantation in acute
    leukemia. UCLA bone marrow transplantation team. Lancet, 2, 1197.
2. Thomas, E.D., Buckner, C.D., Banaji, M., Clift, R.A., Fefer, A.,
    Flournoy, N., Goodell, B.W., Hickman, R.D., Lerner, K.G., Neiman,
    P.E., Sale, G.E., Sanders, J.E., Singer, J., Stevens, M., Storb, R.
    and Weiden, P.L. (1977): One hundred patients with acute leukemia
    treated with chemotherapy, total body irradiation and allogeneic
    marrow transplantation. Blood, 49, 511-533.
3. Bone marrow transplantation. Editorial 1978. Lancet, 1, 859-861.
4. Thomas, E.D., Bryant, J.I., Buckner, C.D., Clift, R.A., Fefer, A.,
    Johnson, F.L., Neiman, P., Ramberg, R.E. and Storb, R. (1972): Leu-
    kaemic transformation of engrafted human marrow cells in vivo.
    Lancet, 1, 1310-1313.
5. Gale, R.P. (1976): Report at the Annual Meeting of the International
    Cooperative Group for BMT in Man, Washington D.C., August 1976.
6. Fefer, A., Buckner, C.D., Thomas, E.D., Cheever, M.A., Clift, R.A.,
    Glucksberg, H., Neiman, P.E. and Storb, R. (1977): Course of hema-
    tologic neoplasia with transplantation of marrow from identical
    twins. New Engl. J. Med., 297, 146-148.
7. Bortin, M.M. and Rimm, A.A. for the Advisory Committee of the In-
    ternational BMT Registry (1978): Bone marrow transplantation for
    acute myeloblastic leukemia. J. Amer. med. Ass., in press.

AUTOLOGOUS BONE MARROW TRANSPLANTATION IN ACUTE LEUKEMIA: A REVIEW[x]

U.W. Schaefer, J.H. Beyer, W.R. Boecker, M.R. Nowrousian,
S. Oehl, C.G. Schmidt, E. Scherer, G. Schmitt, E. Haralam-
bie, G. Linzenmeier, E. Hierholzer, E. Kuwert, W. Luboldt,
L. Gerhard, L.D. Leder, V. Reinhardt, C. Stambolis and D.
Hantschke

Westdeutsches Tumorzentrum, Universitätsklinikum der Gesamt-
hochschule Essen, Federal Republic of Germany

SUMMARY

Hemopoietic stem cells of human bone marrow can be cryopreserved without marked loss of proliferative capacity. Stem cell recovery after
freezing and thawing is significantly influenced by the osmotic characteristics of the cryoprotectants. Osmotic shock after thawing can be
avoided by adequate resuspension techniques.

It has been shown by several authors that cryopreserved autologous bone marrow can be safely infused into patients. However, the
effectiveness of autotransplantations is difficult to assess because
there are no genetic markers to prove a take of an autologous transplant. In a few patients suffering from a blast crisis of CML or from
acute leukemia, transplantations of cryopreserved bone marrow have been
performed after a lethal conditioning regimen. These data are promising,
but it is necessary to investigate more intensively the negative influences of prolonged chemotherapy on the transplantation potential of
the marrow to be cryopreserved.

Several groups have shown that bone marrow stem cells of
mice (1-6), dogs (7-12), monkeys (4,13-15) and man (11,16-
25) can be successfully cryopreserved for prolonged periods.
Stem cell viability in frozen marrow has been investigated
in vivo and in vitro using a variety of techniques.

Quantitative information on stem cell recovery and differentiation can be obtained by transplantation studies in
lethally irradiated recipients by the spleen colony technique (CFU-S), the agar culture technique (CFU-C) and the
diffusion chamber method. Among the agents protecting cells
against freezing damage two different classes have been
described. There are substances (DMSO, glycerol) which provide an intracellular cryoprotection and others which cannot
permeate the cell membrane (PVP, hydroxyethyl starch).

Advances in our understanding of the biological characteristics have led to the conclusion that osmolarity signi-

[x]Supported by Landesamt für Forschung des Landes Nordrhein-Westfalen,
Düsseldorf.

ficantly influences stem cell recovery after freezing and thawing. As the osmolarity of the intracellular cryoprotectives DMSO and glycerol is very high, a rapid adaptation to the physiologic situation causes an osmotic shock. The osmotic stress depends on the degree and duration of the osmotic pressure at the cell membrane. Therefore, in the case of glycerol, which penetrates the cell membrane slowly, marked osmotic problems can be expected.

In contrast to rapid resuspension or immediate injection as used by other investigators we introduced a stepwise dilution technique to remove glycerol or DMSO slowly from the thawed cells, a technique which ameliorates the osmotic gradient at the cell membrane. The superiority of the stepwise dilution technique in the case of intracellular protectants could be shown by us in mice, monkeys and man (26-32). In these species stem cells could be preserved without significant loss of viability. More recently we and others have described that in complete remission of acute leukemia, marrow can also be preserved without significant loss of CFU-C viability (25, 33-34).

CLINICAL TRIALS

Due to numerous reports of successful allogeneic marrow grafting there is renewed interest in bone marrow autotransplantation. When autologous bone marrow is the source of stem cells, graft rejection and GVH disease do not occur. Therefore autologous bone marrow transplantation may provide an approach to treat patients with malignant disease when conventional therapy has failed. The aim is to improve hematologic recovery after aggressive chemo- or radiotherapy, allowing a dose escalation of the therapy and more effective tumor eradication.

Beneficial effects of bone marrow autografts in cancer patients have been described (35-42). But evaluation of the published data must be done very critically. By current standards the doses of chemotherapy or radiotherapy, the cryopreservation methods and the viability assays were often not optimal. An early hematopoietic recovery does not necessarily indicate a take of the transplant. As cytogenetic markers are not available in the autologous situation, a spontaneous recovery of the autochthonous cell population surviving the cytotoxic treatment cannot be excluded.

In recent studies the effect of cryopreserved autologous marrow in patients suffering from blast crisis of chronic myelocytic leukemia (CML) or from acute leukemia has been evaluated.

The Seattle group has treated 7 patients with blast crisis of CML with intensive chemoradiotherapy followed by autotransplantation of bone marrow which was harvested and frozen in 10% DMSO during the chronic phase of the disease (43). The storage time varied from 8 to 32 months, the dose of nucleated cells grafted from 15 to 313 x 10^9. All patients were prepared with cyclophosphamide (120 mg/kg) plus

1000 rad of total body irradiation (TBI) before infusion of stored marrow. Two patients failed to achieve marrow repopulation, 3 patients had partial marrow recovery. Two patients achieved prompt and complete reestablishment of the chronic phase of CML, one died on day 72 with fungal pneumonitis and one developed blastic transformation within 4 months.

The Los Angeles group treated one patient in blast crisis with daunomycin and fractionated total body irradiation and chronic phase bone marrow cryopreserved 9 months earlier (44). The patient had evidence of transient autograft function and died 88 days after transplantation. Goldman who presents his data during this congress, transfused buffy coat cells harvested in the chronic phase and cryopreserved in DMSO to blast crisis CML patients after pretreatment with chemotherapy alone (45).

In acute leukemia an increasing number of autotransplantations have been performed. Bull et al. reported 3 patients treated with polychemotherapy (BACT) followed by autotransplantation (46). There was no restoration of normal hemopoiesis and in 2 cases leukemia reoccurred. One might assume that the transplant contained many leukemic cells. The marrow was cryopreserved in remission but the interval from harvesting to relapse was short.

Gorin could induce remissions by grafting preserved autologous marrow in patients with acute leukemia pretreated with a high dose combination chemotherapy. The author reports his results during this congress (47).

Hellriegel et al. transfused autologous remission marrow preserved in DMSO to a patient with acute promyelocytic leukemia who was pretreated with polychemotherapy (48). A remission of 3 months could be achieved.

Dicke et al. performed autotransplantations in 14 patients with acute leukemia using a lethal conditioning regimen including TBI (960 rad) and piperazinedione (50 mg/m^2) (49). The marrow was harvested during remission and fractionated by the albumin gradient technique in order to attempt a separation of normal and leukemic cells. The marrow was frozen in 10% DMSO and stored for 5-30 months. The number of CFU-C per 10^5 cells transplanted varied from 1 to 30, whereas the grafted cell numbers varied from 8 x 10^6 to 3 x 10^8 per kg body weight (b.w.). In 10 out of 14 cases signs of hematologic recovery were observed. Five of the 10 patients achieved complete hematologic reconstitution. The duration of complete remission ranged from 2 to more than 9 months. At present 2 patients are alive and in complete remission 2+ and 9+ months after transplantation. The causes of death were recurrence of leukemia (2 patients), infections (6 patients) and cardiotoxicity (4 patients) due to anthracycline treatment.

Our group in Essen performed one autotransplantation after lethal conditioning with chemotherapy and TBI. The patient was a 38 year old man suffering from acute myelocytic leukemia. With daunomycin and cytosine arabinoside complete remission could be induced. The remission was maintained by cytosine arabinoside (200 mg/m^2/d x 5 d i.v. every 4 weeks); in addition, a second drug was given which alternated every 4 weeks (thioguanine, cyclophosphamide, CCNU, daunomycin). The marrow was harvested during the first remission after one year of maintenance therapy, 6 weeks after the last chemotherapy course. The interval from cryopreservation to the first relapse was 6 months. The marrow was frozen in 10% DMSO and kept in liquid nitrogen for 15 months. The retransfusion was performed during the second relapse when the disease appeared to be resistant to chemotherapy. The conditioning regimen was the same as in allogeneic bone marrow transplantation. We administered 2 x 50 mg/kg b.w. cyclophosphamide and 860 rad TBI (linear accelerator, 15 rad/min). Twenty-four hours after irradiation the marrow was thawed, diluted according to our method, centrifuged, filtrated and transfused intravenously. 2 x 10^8 nucleated cells per kg b.w. containing approximately 30,000 CFU-C per kg b.w. were administered. Pre- and post-transplantation care was performed under gnotobiotic conditions. The clinical condition of the patient improved dramatically. Two weeks after transplantation the peripheral counts of leukocytes and platelets started to rise and reticulocytes appeared. The maximum leukocyte count of 2,800/mm^3 was reached after 5 weeks. Later the peripheral cell counts dropped again and remained below normal. Regular bone marrow biopsies demonstrated a very good repopulation of the marrow space. The lymphocyte response to PHA increased from 10% to 60% of a normal control. During the third month the marrow cellularity decreased slowly but improved slightly again when corticosteroid therapy was initiated. 145 days after transplantation the patient died pancytopenic from recurrent infections and cerebral bleeding. The post mortem histology revealed an almost normal cellularity. All bone marrow cell classes were present. There was no evidence of a leukemia relapse.

DISCUSSION

The transfusion of cryopreserved autologous remission marrow deserves renewed interest, especially since it has been shown in animal models that leukemic cells may be eliminated from the graft by immunologic means (50). Early trials provided evidence that cryopreserved autologous bone marrow could be infused safely. Better understanding of the cryopreservation process and of the osmotic problems in the post-thawing phase have led to technologic improvements. Marrow culture techniques allow to measure quantitatively the proliferative capacity of preserved marrow in vitro. Progress in pharmacology of antineoplastic drugs and more refined irradiation regimens encourage us to reinvestigate autologous bone marrow transplantation after superaggressive cancerostatic therapy.

Although several authors reported that autotransplantation appeared to reduce the period of granulocytopenia fol-

lowing high-dose chemotherapy, the contribution of autografting is difficult to analyse. In the autologous situation there is no genetic marker to prove the take of a
frozen transplant. Marrow recovery may occur in a similar
pattern without marrow grafting. Therefore, approaches
which include a supralethal pretreatment regimen using
high-dose chemotherapy and TBI are of great interest. Dicke
showed that cryopreserved autografts in acute leukemia can
restore hematopoiesis and induce long-term remissions. Observations of Hellman and co-workers in mice (51) and of
Lohrmann in man (52) demonstrate that the hematopoietic
capacity might be disturbed significantly and for a long
time when repeated courses of chemotherapy have been administered. Our own data indicate that the transplantation
potential of frozen remission marrow might be impaired in
spite of prompt take and normal proliferation of the cells
to be grafted in the agar assay and in the diffusion chamber. It could be speculated that the prolonged chemotherapy,
which our patient received before the marrow was cryopreserved, perturbated self-reproduction and differentiation
potential of the marrow stem cells. We investigated the
CFU-C content of the marrow in a number of remission patients. There is indication that aggressive maintenance
therapy induces a steady decrease of the CFU-C numbers.
These data will be published elsewhere. The effect of prolonged chemotherapy on the transplantation potential,
methods to recognize and separate residual leukemic cells
from the transplant and new concepts of chemoradiotherapy
for eradication of malignant cells are the most challenging
aspects in autologous bone marrow transplantation.

REFERENCES

1. Ashwood-Smith, M.J. (1961): Preservation of mouse bone marrow at
    -79°C with dimethyl sulphoxide. Nature (Lond.), 190, 1204-1205.
2. Lewis, J.P. and Trobaugh Jr, F.E. (1964): The assay of the trans-
    plantation potential of fresh and stored bone marrow by two in-
    vivo systems. Ann. N.Y. Acad. Sci., 114, 677-685.
3. Leibo, S.P., Farnes, M.P., Albala, M. and Trobaugh Jr, F.E. (1964):
    Transplantation potential of fresh and stored hematopoietic tissue
    as estimated by standard in-vitro techniques. Ann. N.Y. Acad. Sci.,
    114, 701-713.
4. Van Putten, L.M. (1965): Quantitative aspects of the storage of
    bone marrow cells for transplantation. Europ. J. Cancer, 1, 15-22.
5. Lewis, J.P., Passovoy, M. and Trobaugh Jr, F.E. (1966): The trans-
    plantation efficiency of marrow cooled to -100°C at 2°C per minute.
    Cryobiology, 3, 47-52.
6. Leibo, S.P., Farrant, J., Mazur, P., Hanna Jr, M.G. and Smith,
    L.H. (1970): Effects of freezing on marrow stem cell suspensions:
    interactions of cooling and warming rates in the presence of PVP,
    sucrose, or glycerol. Cryobiology, 6, 315-332.
7. Mannick, J.A., Lochte Jr, H.L., Thomas, E.D. and Ferrebee, J.W.
    (1960): In vitro and in vivo assessment of the viability of dog
    marrow after storage. Blood, 15, 517-524.
8. Cavins, J.A., Kasakura, S., Thomas, E.D. and Ferrebee, J.W. (1962):

Recovery of lethally irradiated dogs following infusion of autologous marrow stored at low temperature in dimethylsulphoxide. Blood, 20, 730-734.

9. Storb, R., Epstein, R.B., Le Blond, R.F., Rudolph, R.H. and Thomas, E.D. (1969): Transplantation of allogeneic canine bone marrow stored at -80°C in dimethyl sulfoxide. Blood, 33, 918-923.

10. Bruch, C., Herbst, E., Calvo, W., Huget, P., Flad, H.D. and Fliedner, T.M. (1973): Freezing of blood leucocytes for transplantation into lethally irradiated dogs. In: La cryoconservation des cellules normales et néoplasiques / The cryopreservation of normal and neoplastic cells. Proceedings of the International Conference held at Villejuif, France, June 30, 1973, pp. 51-62. Editors: R.S. Weiner, R.K. Oldham and L. Schwarzenberg. Editions INSERM, Paris.

11. Debelak-Fehir, K.M., Bennett, B.T. and Epstein, R.B. (1974): Transplantation potential of fresh and cryopreserved peripheral blood stem cells in man and dog. In: Abstracts of the 5th International Congress of the Transplantation Society, Jerusalem, Israel, August 25-30, 1974, p. 200.

12. Gorin, N.C., Herzig, G., Bull, M.I. and Graw Jr, R.G. (1978): Long-term perservation of bone marrow and stem cell pool in dogs. Blood, 51, 257-265.

13. Van Putten, L.M., Van Bekkum, D.W. and Dicke, K.A. (1969): The storage of primate bone marrow for homologous transplantation. In: Annual Report, 1968, p. 62. Radiobiological Institute, Institute for Experimental Gerontology, and Primate Center, TNO, Rijswijk.

14. Buckner, C.D., Storb, R., Dillingham, L.A. and Thomas, E.D. (1970): Low temperature preservation of monkey marrow in dimethyl sulfoxide. Cryobiology, 7, 136-140.

15. Merritt, C.B., Darrow, C.C., Vaal, L., Herzig, G.P. and Rogentine Jr, G.N. (1973): Rescue of rhesus monkeys from acute lethal graft-versus-host disease using cyclophosphamide and frozen autologous bone marrow. Transplantation, 15, 154-159.

16. Lochte Jr, H.L., Ferrebee, J.W. and Thomas, E.D. (1959): In vitro studies on the preservation of marrow cells in glycerol at low temperatures. J. Lab. clin. Med., 53, 117-126.

17. Pyle, H.M. and Boyer, H.F. (1964): Factors influencing the post-storage viability of human bone marrow. Ann. N.Y. Acad. Sci., 114, 686-694.

18. Malinin, T.I., Pegg, D.E., Perry, V.P. and Brodine, C.E. (1970): Long-term storage of bone marrow cells at liquid nitrogen and dry ice temperatures. Cryobiology, 7, 65-69.

19. Sultan, C. and Soulas, S. (1970): Technique de congélation de moëlles humaines en vue d'autogreffe. Résultats préliminaires. Path. et Biol., 18, 1097-1100.

20. Berthier, R. and Marcille, G. (1972): Agar colony formation as a measure of viability for frozen bone marrow cells. In: In vitro culture of hemopoietic cells. Proceedings of a Workshop/Symposium, Rijswijk, 1971, pp. 377-385. Editors: D.W. Van Bekkum and K.A. Dicke. Radiobiological Institute TNO, Rijswijk.

21. Collmann, H. and Boll, I. (1972): Untersuchungen zur Proliferationskinetik der Erythropoese von gefrierkonserviertem Knochenmark in vitro. Blut, 25, 265-273.

22. Adamson, J.W. and Storb, R. (1972): The proliferative potential of frozen stored human marrow cells, Transplantation, 14, 490-494.

23. Mosimann, W., Furlan, M., Beck, E.A. and Bucher, U. (1972): Zellkonservierung durch Tiefkühlung, mit besonderer Berücksichtigung des Knochenmarks. Schweiz. med. Wschr., 102, 1600-1602.

24. Gray, J.L. and Robinson, W.A. (1973): In vitro colony formation by human bone marrow cells after freezing. J. Lab. clin. Med., 81, 317-322.

25. Netzel, B., Haas, R.J., Janka, G.E. and Thierfelder, S. (1978): Viability of stem cells (CFU-C) after long term cryopreservation of bone marrow cells from normal adults and children with acute lymphoblastic leukemia in remission. In: Cell-separation and cryobiology. Selected papers of an International Symposium in Vienna, 9-12 November 1977, pp. 255-258. Editors: H. Rainer, H. Borberg, J.M. Mishler and U.W. Schaefer. Schattauer, Stuttgart, New York.

26. Schaefer, U.W., Dicke, K.A. and Klein, J.C. (1972): In vitro and in vivo studies with stored bone marrow cells of mouse and monkey. In: In vitro culture of hemopoietic cells. Proceedings of a Workshop/Symposium, Rijswick, 1971, pp. 187-196. Editors: D.W. Van Bekkum and K.A. Dicke. Radiobiological Institute TNO, Rijswijk.

27. Schaefer, U.W., Dicke, K.A. and Van Bekkum, D.W. (1972): Recovery of haemopoiesis in lethally irradiated monkeys by frozen allogeneic bone marrow grafts. Rev. europ. Etud. clin. biol., 17, 483-488.

28. Schaefer, U.W. and Dicke, K.A. (1972): Konservierung von Knochenmark. Verh. dtsch. Ges. inn. Med., 78, 1601-1603.

29. Schaefer, U.W. and Dicke, K.A. (1973): Preservation of haemopoietic stem cells. Transplantation potential and CFU-C activity of frozen marrow tested in mice, monkeys and man. In: La cryoconservation des cellules normales et néoplasiques / The cryopreservation of normal and neoplastic cells. Proceedings of the International Conference held at Villejuif, France, June 30, 1973, pp. 63-69. Editors: R.S. Weiner, R.K. Oldham and L. Schwarzenberg. Editions INSERM, Paris.

30. Schaefer, U.W., Schmidt, C.G., Dicke, K.A., Van Bekkum, D.W. and Schmitt, G. (1975): Konservierung von hämopoetischen Stammzellen. Z. Krebsforsch., 83, 285-291.

31. Schaefer, U.W., Öhl, S. and Nowrousian, M.R. (1977): Bestimmung der zytopoetischen Kapazität von kryopräserviertem menschlichem Knochenmark in vitro (Agarkultur) und in vivo (Diffusionskammer). Verh. dtsch. Ges. inn. Med., 83, 1230-1231.

32. Schaefer, U.W., Nowrousian, M.R., Öhl, S. and Schmidt, C.G. (1978): Cryopreservation of bone marrow. In: Cell-separation and cryobiology. Selected papers of an International Symposium in Vienna, 9-12 November, 1977, pp. 243-254. Editors: H. Rainer, H. Borberg, J.M. Mishler and U.W. Schaefer. Schattauer, Stuttgart, New York.

33. Ragab, A.H., Gilkerson, E. and Choi, S.C. (1974): The cryopreservation of colony-forming cells from the bone marrow of children with acute lymphocytic leukemia. Cancer Res., 34, 942-946.

34. Balkwill, F., Pindar, A. and Crowther, D. (1974): Factors influencing microculture of leukaemia cells. Nature (Lond.), 251, 741-742.

35. Thomas, E.D., Lochte Jr, H.L., Lu, W.C. and Ferrebee, J.W. (1957): Intravenous infusion of bone marrow in patients receiving radiation and chemotherapy. New Engl. J. Med., 257, 491-496.

36. Pegg, D.E., Humble, J.G. and Newton, K.A. (1962): The clinical application of bone marrow grafting. Brit. J. Cancer, 16, 417-435.

37. Lawrik, S. (1970): Langzeitkonservierung von Knochenmark im gefrorenen Zustand bei -196°C. Folia haemat. (Lpz.), 94, 261-263.
38. Polese, E., Massenti, S. and Rossi-Torelli, M. (1970): Efficacia del midollo autologo conservato su pazienti sottoposti a trattamento terapeutico mielodepressivo. Minerva med., 61, 4159-4162.
39. Buckner, C.D., Rudolph, R.H., Fefer, A., Clift, R.A., Epstein, R.B., Funk, D.D., Neiman, P.E., Slichter, S.J., Storb, R. and Thomas, E.D. (1972): High-dose cyclophosphamide therapy for malignant disease. Toxicity, tumor response, and the effects of stored autologous marrow. Cancer (Philad.), 29, 357-365.
40. Appelbaum, F., Gratwohl, A., Ziegler, J.L., Levine, A.S. and Deisseroth, A. (1977): Autologous bone marrow infusions and acceleration of hematopoietic recovery following ablative chemotherapy in man. Exp. Hemat., 5, Suppl. 2, 104.
41. Weiner, R.S. (1977): Autologous bone marrow transplantation in man: laboratory and clinical studies. Exp. Hemat., 5, Suppl. 2, 104.
42. Kühböck, J., Karrer, K. and Mannheimer, E. (1978): Haematological observations on patients after re-infusion of frozen stored bone marrow. In: Cell-separation and cryobiology. Selected papers of an International Symposium in Vienna, 9-12 November, 1977, pp. 297-300. Editors: H. Rainer, H. Borberg, J.M. Mishler and U.W. Schaefer. Schattauer, Stuttgart, New York.
43. Buckner, C.D., Stewart, P., Clift, R.A., Fefer, A., Neiman, P.E., Singer, J., Storb, R. and Thomas, E.D. (1978): Treatment of blastic transformation of chronic granulocytic leukemia by chemotherapy, total body irradiation and infusion of cryopreserved autologous marrow. Exp. Hemat., 6, 96-109.
44. Graze, P.R. and Gale, R.P. (1978): Autotransplantation for leukemia and solid tumors. Transplant. Proc., 10, 177-184.
45. Goldman, J.M. (1979): New approaches to the treatment of acute myeloid leukaemia and chronic granulocytic leukaemia in transformation. This volume.
46. Bull, M.I., Appelbaum, F.R., Fay, J.W. et al. (1976): Exp. Hemat., 4, Suppl., 146: Cit. Graze and Gale (44).
47. Gorin, N.C. (1979): Critical evaluation of the conditioning regimen and autologous bone marrow transplantation in acute leukaemia. This volume.
48. Hellriegel, K.P., Hirschmann, W.D., Gauwerky, C., Gerecke, D., Borberg, H. and Gross, R. (1978): Autologous bone marrow transplantation in acute leukemia. In: Cell-separation and cryobiology. Selected papers of an International Symposium in Vienna, 9-12 November, 1977, pp. 335-339. Editors: H. Rainer, H. Borberg, J.M. Mishler and U.W. Schaefer. Schattauer, Stuttgart, New York.
49. Dicke, K.A., Zander, A., McCredie, K.B., Spitzer, G., Verma, D.S. and Vellekoop, L. (1978): Autologous bone marrow transplantation in relapsed adult acute leukemia. Exp. Hemat., 6, Suppl. 3, 8.
50. Thierfelder, S., Rodt, H. and Netzel, B. (1977): Transplantation of syngeneic bone marrow incubated with leucocyte antibodies. I. Suppression of lymphatic leukemia of syngeneic donor mice. Transplantation, 23, 459-563.
51. Hellman, S., Botnick, L.E., Hannon, E.C. and Vigneulle, R.M. (1978): Proliferative capacity of murine hematopoietic stem cells. Proc. nat. Acad. Sci. (Wash.), 75, 490-494.

52. Lohrmann, H.P., Schreml, W., Fliedner, T.M. and Heimpel, H. (1978): Reaction of human granulopoiesis to high-dose cyclophosphamide therapy. Exp. Hemat., 6, Suppl. 3, 49.

CRYOPRESERVATION OF HUMAN BONE MARROW WITH A VIEW TO AUTOL-
OGOUS BONE MARROW TRANSPLANTATION

P. Herve, E. Tamayo, C. Coffe, R. Lenus and A. Peters

Blood Transfusion Center, Besancon, France

SUMMARY

Autologous bone marrow transplantation in which the patient's own bone
marrow cells are cryopreserved in liquid nitrogen and then reinfused
after adminstration of chemotherapy offers a method by which bone marrow suppression may be avoided.
    Marrow cells obtained by multiple punctures are enriched by use
of a blood separator (Haemonetics Model 30). The buffy coat is collected in a transfer bag containing plasma/ACD. Before freezing, the cell
concentration must be adjusted to 5 x 10^6/ml. DMSO is added slowly to
a final concentration of 10%. The cell suspension is transferred in
Teflon-Kapton bags (frozen volume is 100 ml) and the freezing rate is
2°C/min down to -6°C, then 10°C/min to -40°C, and then 5°C/min to
-140°C (we use an electronic freezer provided with a programmer). The
bag is stored in liquid nitrogen. After thawing (42°C-45°C), the cells
are diluted in a stepwise manner. The osmolarity of the dilution media
must be chosen according to the osmotic stress borne by the cells when
the DMSO is eliminated. We use enriched media whose osmolarity is
progressively decreased. Three dilution solutions are used and after
the third, the marrow cells are suspended in an iso-osmolar medium
before infusion.
    We have tested the viability of stem cells before and after freez-
ing using the ability of colony-forming cells to form colonies in agar.
We have obtained a CFC recovery of about 82%.

The establishment of a chemotherapy protocol for malignant
hemopathies, as for solid tumors, must take into account
the close relationship that exists between dosage and medullary toxicity. The post chemotherapy bone marrow failures
are sometimes of such gravity (due especially to infectious
complications) that one hesitates to use strong doses of
antineoplastic drugs. Nevertheless, it is well known that
complete remission is proportional to the intensity of the
iatrogenic bone marrow failures. For the acute leukemias,
chemotherapy is not successful, particularly for the destruction of malignant cells situated in the central nervous
system. Total body irradiation might complete the antineoplastic effects of chemotherapy in these areas. But this
cannot be undertaken without hematological reanimation associated with a bone marrow graft.

With the progress seen in recent years in cryobiology, it has become apparent that the application of low temperatures for the preservation of blood cells, and more recently hemopoietic stem cells, could permit an approach to hematological reanimation from a different view point. In theory, the principle of autologous marrow grafts is simple. Bone marrow which must meet all criteria for normality, is taken during complete remission. The marrow cells are cryopreserved until the relapse of the hemopathy, or the appearance of the metastatic dissemination phase of a solid tumor, then reinjected after supralethal body irradiation. The survival of the patient depends closely upon the quantity and the proliferative capacity of the injected CFU-C.

MATERIALS AND METHODS

Bone marrow aspiration

Marrow cells are obtained from the anterior and posterior iliac crests by multiple punctures with Jamshidi needles (Kormed Inc., Minneapolis, USA). The syringes must be heparinized. The bone marrow is placed in several plastic bags (TA$_2$, Fenwal) containing an anticoagulant solution (RPMI with 2400 units of preservative free heparin). In most cases the total volume aspirated was 800 to 900 ml.

Bone marrow concentration

The marrow cells are enriched with a blood separator (Haemonetics Model 30) using a technique inspired by Weiner (8) (Fig. 1).
After aspiration, all of the cells in the plastic bags are pooled and placed in a large bag (TA$_{10}$, Fenwal), which is then connected to the cell separator using the standard donor set-up. After the first cycle, the remaining blood and plasma is returned to the 'return bag'. The procedure is repeated until the aspirate has passed through the bowl at least 2 or 3 times using the 225-ml bowl (we intend to use in future the 100-ml bowl, which is now available). The anticoagulant solution is ACD/saline/heparin. The filling rate of the bowl is 60 ml/min and the setting time of the buffy coat is 1 min. The buffy coat is collected in a 300-ml transfer bag containing plasma and ACD.

Bone marrow freezing and storage

The cellular concentration before freezing is about 5×10^6/ml. Dimethylsulfoxide (DMSO) is added very slowly to a final concentration of 10% in plasma. After 10-min incubation in melting ice, the cell suspension is dispensed into several plastic bags (the frozen volume in each bag is 100 ml to 150 ml). The containers used are Teflon-Kapton bags (Gambro Dialysatoren, Hechingen, Germany) with a holder adapted to ensure a homogeneous distribution of the solution

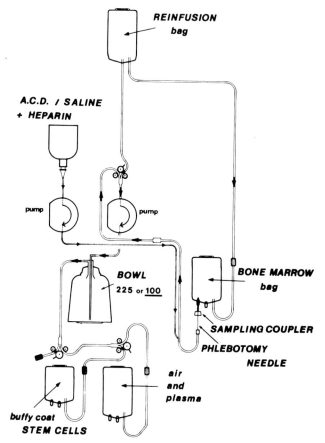

Fig. 1. Semicontinuous flow centrifugation for the concentration of stem cells.

to be frozen.

The machine we use is an electronic freezer provided with a programmer (Nicool, supplied by l'Air liquide). The probe is always placed in a reference bag containing an identical solution (plasma and DMSO). Marrow cells are frozen at a controlled rate of 2°C/min to -6°C, then at 1°C/min to -40°C and then at 5°C/min to -140°C. At the time of supercooling, a temperature of -19°C in the freezing chamber is required to obtain a minimum of heat of fusion. The rewarming rate at room temperature is so fast that it is necessary to transfer the bags extremely rapidly to the liquid nitrogen for storage.

Bone marrow thawing and dilution

Thawing must be done rapidly at +40°C in a water bath. The method of dilution is carried out in a stepwise fashion. The osmolarity of the dilution media is chosen according to the osmotic stress borne by the cells. We use enriched media that permit a progressive decrease of the osmolarity:

sol. 1 - Robinson medium - saline - citrate - DNAse (450 mOs); sol. 2 - Robinson medium - hypertonic saline 1.75% (600 mOs); sol. 3 - Robinson medium - distilled water - ACD (220 mOs).

Marrow cells are centrifuged once to remove most of the DMSO. After the third dilution the cells are suspended in an iso-osmolar medium and they are ready for infusion.

In vitro tests to judge the efficiency of the method

The viability of myelocytic progenitor cells is assessed both in fresh specimens and in aliquots of cryopreserved specimens by bone marrow colony formation in culture, as reported by Robinson and Pike (3). We have used the 2-layer agar technique.

The feeder layer (see below) contains blood leukocytes, as the source of colony-stimulating factor. Bone marrow cells (2×10^5 cells) are placed in this upper layer. The Petri dishes are incubated at $37^{o}C$ in a humid atmosphere of 7% carbon dioxide. CFU-C are counted after incubation for 9-12 days. Morphological studies on the primitive cells are performed under optical microscope.

RESULTS

Morphological study

The morphology of the marrow cells before and after cryo-preservation was compared in all samples. Prior to freezing 45-70% of the cells were myeloid cells. After freezing and thawing less than 10% of the cells were myeloid and 90% of the cells consisted of mononuclear cells and nucleated red cells. By microscopy, few structural modifications in the primitive cells (myeloblast, proerythroblast) were seen. In some cases, the modifications observed were either cyto-plasmic vacuoles or excrescences from the membrane.

In vitro study of colony formation

The relative CFU-C recovery after freezing is calculated according to the following formula:

$$\text{CFU-C recovery} = \frac{\text{CFU-C/2} \times 10^5 \text{ nucleated cells after freezing}}{\text{CFU-C/2} \times 10^5 \text{ nucleated cells before freezing}} \times 100$$

In 20 experiments, the mean CFU-C recovery was about 82% (Fig. 2).

There was no significant difference between the per-centage of CFU-C recovery at one week or one month. It, therefore, seems that the greatest loss of stem cells occurred in the process of cryopreservation itself.

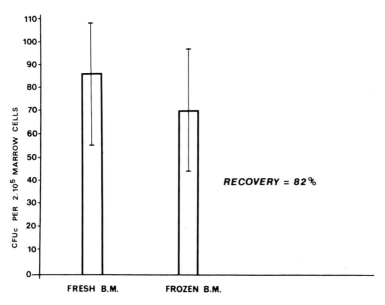

Fig. 2. Survival of CFU-C in frozen human bone marrow.

DISCUSSION

The efficiency of a freezing method and its capacity to be reproduced depend very closely on all the chosen parameters and it is necessary to respect each one during the procedure. Several cryoprotectors have been proposed in the past for freezing bone marrow (2,5,6). The cryoprotector most often employed was DMSO. The concentration used varied between 8 and 12%. Overall, the results were in favor of a final concentration of 10%. The cell viability was in close relation to the osmolarity phenomenon. The 10% DMSO solution presented optimal osmolarity, which justified the precautions when adding the cryoprotector to the cell suspension. Its toxicity for humans remains a preoccupation. For this reason we preferred to wash the thawed bone marrow to eliminate the majority of DMSO. It would be beneficial to use a non-toxic cryoprotector during bone marrow freezing. This would allow the infusion of thawed bone marrow without prior washing (the washing step may be the origin of the loss of cells).
    We studied the action of glycerol at concentrations of 6-10%. Even without washing we have observed after thawing a greater number of cellular aggregates. The perfection of more sophisticated techniques to purify cell populations for freezing will facilitate the comparative studies between different cryoprotectors (cellular heterogeneity of a marrow suspension is often the origin of difficulties in interpreting the results obtained when comparing cryoprotectors). Results from the experiments using glycerol merit further investigation in combination with purification methods that eliminate platelets and granulocytes.

Polyethyleneoxide (4) seems to present several advantages in cryobiology: a cryoprotector effect and the absence of human toxicity. The prospects offered by this cryoprotector merit further investigation. In the future, the principal improvement in the freezing of stem cells must be the utilization of a cryoprotector that avoids the washing step.

The great value of the purification method involving semicontinuous flow centrifugation is the possibility of freezing the bone marrow in small volumes and eliminating most of the red blood cells, platelets and many granulocytes (these cells contribute to severe clumping resulting in cell loss upon thawing). It is necessary to use bags very resistant to low temperature. Using Gambro bags there is less than 1% rupture of the bags during thawing. This quality is essential if human bone marrow is being preserved for grafting. Even though the parameters for the freezing technique are now established the thawing dilution stage remains the most delicate and influences the outcome. The stepwise procedure still gives the best results. It is only after these preparatory steps have been mastered that autologous transplantation may be attempted.

It is necessary to study the repopulation kinetics of the marrow areas by the thawed stem cells and to define the role of this technique in the treatment of acute leukemias. Only random studies will permit a confirmation of interest in this method. Malignant hemopathies such as acute myeloid leukemia, acute T lymphoblastic leukemia, chronic myeloid leukemia (1,7) were the first conditions proposed for autologous grafts. The time of marrow removal during the course of the disease seems to be a determining factor. For example, how far from complete remission should it be performed? Should it be as soon as possible or after several treatments? The marrow should not be taken until after one evaluation of stem cell proliferation using the in vitro colony-formation technique. The criteria for complete remission are essentially defined by a cytological study of the bone marrow. There is a risk of taking and conserving a clone of malignant cells that may be present as dormant cells in the sample and which may be resistant to freezing. This might be a reason for a relapse seen after the autologous graft.

As for the marrow graft itself, it is usually accepted that the number of nucleated cells to be infused must be at least 1×10^8 cells/kg. If the graft is done with a purified suspension of mononuclear cells, the number to be used is questionable. It should be calculated as a function of the number of CFU-C for 2×10^5 mononuclear cells: i.e., approximately $4-6 \times 10^4$ CFU-C/kg.

There are two fundamentally different situations when autografting can be undertaken. The first is at the moment of relapse after a supralethal treatment by total body irradiation and chemotherapy to induce complete aplasia. Under these conditions autologous bone marrow is thawed and infused (Fig. 3). The second is immediately after complete remission in order to consolidate the result and increase the duration of remission (Fig. 4).

If these studies on autografting of acute leukemias confirm the interest of this procedure, many more situations should become evident. We can cite lymphomas, reticular sarcomas and solid tumors in the initial phase before metastasis. For these diseases, where the changes of conserving a healthy bone marrow are much higher the indication for autologous transplantations are better.

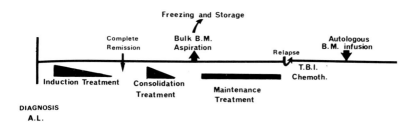

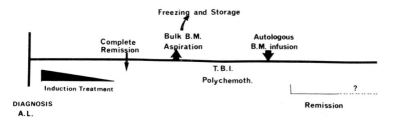

Figs. 3 + 4. Freezing of human bone marrow.

REFERENCES

1. Buckner, C.D., Clift, R.A., Fefer, A., Neiman, P.E., Storb, R. and Thomas, E.D. (1974): Treatment of blastic transformation of chronic granulocytic leukemia by high dose cyclophosphamide total body irradiation and infusion of cryopreserved autologous marrow. Exp. Hemat., 2, 138-146.
2. Malinin, T.I., Pegg, D.E., Perry, V.P. and Brodine, C.E. (1970): Long term storage of bone marrow cells at liquid nitrogen and dry ice temperature. Cryobiology, 7, 65-71.

3. Pike, B.L. and Robinson, W.A. (1970): Human bone marrow colony growth in agar gel. J. cell. Physiol., 76, 77-84.
4. Pushkar, N.S., Shenberg, M.G. and Oboznaya, E.I. (1976): On the mechanism of cryoprotection by polyethylene oxide. Cryobiology, 13, 142-146.
5. Ragab, A.H., Gilkerson, E. and Myers, M. (1977): Factors in the cryopreservation of bone marrow cells from children with acute lymphocytic leukemia. Cryobiology, 14, 125-134.
6. Schaefer, U.W. and Dicke, K.A. (1973): Preservation of haemopoietic stem cells. Transplantation potential and CFU-C activity of frozen marrow tested in mice, monkeys and man. In: Cryopreservation des Cellules Normales et Néoplastiques, pp. 63-68. INSERM Monograph.
7. Tobias, J.S., Weiner, R.S., Griffiths, C.T., Richman, C.M., Parker, L.M. and Yankee, R.A. (1977): Cryopreserved autologous marrow infusion following high dose cancer chemotherapy. Europ. J. Cancer, 13, 269-277.
8. Weiner, R.S., Richman, C.M. and Yankee, R.A. (1977): Semi-continuous flow centrifugation for the pheresis of immunocompetent cells and stem cells. Blood, 49, 391-397.

HIGH DOSE COMBINATION CHEMOTHERAPY (TACC) WITH AND WITHOUT AUTOLOGOUS BONE MARROW TRANSPLANTATION FOR THE TREATMENT OF ACUTE LEUKEMIA, AND OTHER MALIGNANT DISEASES

Kinetics of recovery of hemopoiesis - A preliminary study of 11 cases

N.C. Gorin[1], R. David[1], J. Stachowiak[1], F. Hirsch Marie[1], J.C. Petit[2], J.Y. Muller[3], G. Leblanc[1], Y. Parlier[1], Ch. Salmon[3] and G. Duhamel[1]

[1]Department of Hematology and [2]Laboratoire de Bactériologie, Hôpital Saint-Antoine, and [3]Centre National de Transfusion Sanguine, Etablissement Saint-Antoine, Paris, France

SUMMARY

Eleven patients with drug-resistant tumors (4 solid tumors, 7 acute leukemias) have been treated with a high dose combination chemotherapy regimen (TACC) consisting of: cyclophosphamide 45 mg/kg days 1-4, ARA-C and 6-TG 100 mg/m^2 each q 12 h days 1-4; CCNU 200 mg/m^2 single dose on day 3.

Following chemotherapy, 7 patients (4 solid tumors, 1 AML, 2 acute monoblastic leukemias) received cryopreserved marrow harvested at a time when bone marrow examination was normal. The doses of bone marrow infused ranged from 0.5-2.2 10^8 nucleated bone marrow cells/kg and had been preserved for periods of up to 6 months. Recovery to a WBC count of 1000 mm^{-3} occurred on days 12-19 (median day 17) and recovery to a platelet count of 50,000 mm^{-3} occurred on days 9-28 (median day 15). All 3 patients with acute leukemia went into complete remission (3, 3 and 5 months). One patient with Hodgkin's disease went into complete remission. The other patients went into partial remission.

Four patients (1 ALL, 1 AML, 2 CML in blastic crisis) did not receive autologous marrow after chemotherapy. One patient (ALL) went into a complete remission with a recovery to a WBC count of 1000 mm^{-3} on day 30 and recovery to a platelet count of 50,000 mm^{-3} on day 35. This patient relapsed on day 69. Two other patients recovered a WBC count of 1000 mm^{-3} on days 27 and 28 with 77% and 9% residual circulating leukemic cells. The last patient (CML in blastic crisis) died on day 15 with persisting leukemic proliferation.

These data support the following statements: (1) The TACC high dose combination chemotherapy (a) does not induce irreversible aplasia in leukemic patients; (b) does not eradicate leukemia. (2) Combined with high dose combination chemotherapy, the reinfusion of cryopreserved marrow (a) is beneficial in that it shortens the duration of the aplasia in all patients; (b) provides a sufficient number of normal stem cells to induce a complete remission in acute leukemia, resistant to conventional chemotherapy.

Autologous bone marrow transplantation has been shown to
rescue severe myelosuppression in numerous experimental
models (1,2,5,6,10,16,17,18,20,23). We have recently demonstrated in dogs a 100% preservation of stem cells following
periods of storage for up to 5 months, with an 'optimum'
freezing technique (11).

In man, autologous bone marrow transplantation may be
of benefit in allowing higher dosage and more prolonged
administration of chemotherapy and radiotherapy in responding tumors. It may also be used in an attempt to rescue
graft rejection or severe graft-versus-host disease (GVHD)
after allogeneic transplantation. However, few autologous
bone marrow transplantations have been done in man (3,7,8)
and the viability of the frozen human stem cell is still
questioned.

In 1976, we initiated a therapeutic trial in an attempt
to demonstrate the feasibility of autologous bone marrow
transplantation in man. The purpose was to evaluate its
contribution to the treatment of acute leukemias resistant
to conventional chemotherapy (12) as well as of some other
drug-resistant malignancies that do not have bone marrow
involvement.

Eleven patients received a high dose combination chemotherapy regimen (TACC) slightly modified from the original
BACT (13) generally used as a conditioning regimen for
allogeneic bone marrow transplantation. Of these 11 patients, 7 received cryopreserved autologous marrow, whereas
4 received only supportive care.

MATERIAL AND METHODS

Patients (Table 1)

The patients were divided into 3 groups. Group 1 consisted
of 4 patients with non-curable solid tumors without bone
marrow involvement. These patients received the TACC regimen
followed by the infusion of cryopreserved marrow. Group 2
consisted of 3 patients with acute leukemia in relapse.
These patients received the TACC regimen and cryopreserved
marrow which had been harvested during the first remission
phase. Group 3 consisted of 4 patients with drug-resistant
acute leukemia. These patients received the same high dose
combination chemotherapy regimen without cryopreserved
marrow.

Bone marrow harvesting, freezing and storage

To collect bone marrow cells under general anesthesia, we
used the procedure previously described by Thomas et al.
(21). The nucleated bone marrow cell count was calculated
and corrected for dilution with media and peripheral blood,
using the assumption that the number of nucleated cells
present in excess of the peripheral blood leukocyte count
represents bone marrow cells.

TABLE 1. Distribution of patients

GROUP 1 (SOLID TUMORS)	T	
1 Nasopharyngeal carcinoma		INFUSION OF
1 Rhabdomyosarcoma		
1 Hodgkin's disease		
1 Localized plasmocytoma of the liver		CRYOPRESERVED
	A	
GROUP 2 (ACUTE LEUKEMIAS)		AUTOLOGOUS MARROW
1 AML		
2 Acute monoblastic leukemias		
	C	
GROUP 3 (ACUTE LEUKEMIAS)		
1 ALL		
1 AML		NO AUTOLOGOUS MARROW
2 CML in blastic crisis	C	

The fresh marrow suspension was separated into samples of 100 ml in Hemoflex bags (catalogue No. 7450-2 Union Carbide Corp. Chicago, Ill). Erythrocytes were not removed before freezing. The freezing solution consisting of 20% DMSO and 10% decomplemented human AB serum in TC 199 medium (Gibco Biocult - Glasgow, Scotland, UK) was prepared freshly and added to the bone marrow suspension in equal volume, immediately prior to freezing. Each bag was compressed between 2 flat aluminium plates so that temperature was uniformly distributed. The marrow was frozen in a Cryoson BV-4 biological freezing system (Cryoson, Midden Beemster, Holland), modified to react to the heat of fusion, by increasing the release of nitrogen vapor. The freezing rate was $-1^{o}C/min$ to fusion and then dropped to $-6^{o}C/min$ to $-60^{o}C$ when the bags were transferred to the gas phase of a liquid nitrogen freezer. The bags were stored below $-140^{o}C$ (Fig. 1).

High dose combination chemotherapy (TACC)

The basic 4-day course of TACC consisted of: cyclophosphamide 45 mg/kg day 1-4; ARA-C 100 mg/m^2 q 12 h day 1-4; 6-thioguanine 100 mg/m^2 q 12 h day 1-4; CCNU 200 mg/m^2 day 2.
One patient in Group 1 (rhabdomyosarcoma) received an extended 5-day course of TACC with a total dose of cyclophosphamide 225 mg/kg (18 g), ARA-C and 6-TG 900 mg/m^2, CCNU 200 mg/m^2.

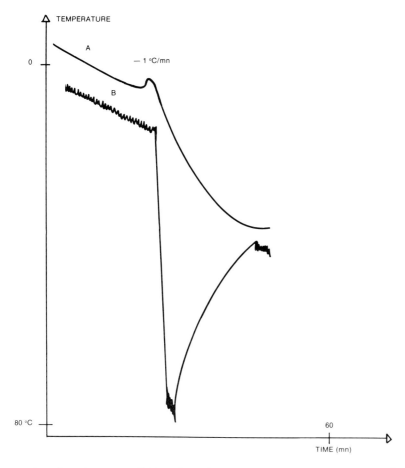

Fig. 1. Diagram of the freezing curves. A: temperature of the sample of bone marrow. B: Temperature inside the freezing chamber.

Autologous engraftment

Frozen marrow was quickly thawed in a water bath at 37°C and infused immediately, with no attempt to remove DMSO or destroyed red cells. Bone marrow was administered by intravenous infusion without filtration, 48 hours after the last dose of cyclophosphamide, and at least 72 hours after CCNU. Two bags of bone marrow were administered simultaneously to avoid renal damage resulting from hemoglobinuria. Hyperdiuresis (4 l/m^2) initially started with the administration of cyclophosphamide, was pursued until the urine cleared. Dexchlorpheniramine maleate was given to counteract the effects of expected histamine release associated with IV DMSO.

Except for the first patient, all patients were treated in a protected environment and received non-absorbable antibiotics for bowel decontamination.

91

During the period of aplasia, the patients were supported with frozen red cells and the platelets were collected with the cell separator (Aminco, Silver Spring, Maryland) to maintain the platelet count above 30,000 mm^{-3}. All blood products were irradiated with 2500 rads. Day 0 is the day of marrow infusion in Groups 1 and 2 and the corresponding day for patients in Group 3.

RESULTS

Except for nausea and vomiting, the TACC regimen was well tolerated in all cases and there was no sign of cardiotoxicity and no hematuria. Two cases of Staphylococcus aureus sepsis developed in Groups 1 and 2, and 3 cases of sepsis (1 Staphylococcus, 1 Escherichia coli, 1 Candida albicans) developed in Group 3. Renal function tests routinely done in all patients did not show any damage in relation to hemoglobinuria. Groups 1 and 2 were similar in terms of hemopoietic reconstitution:

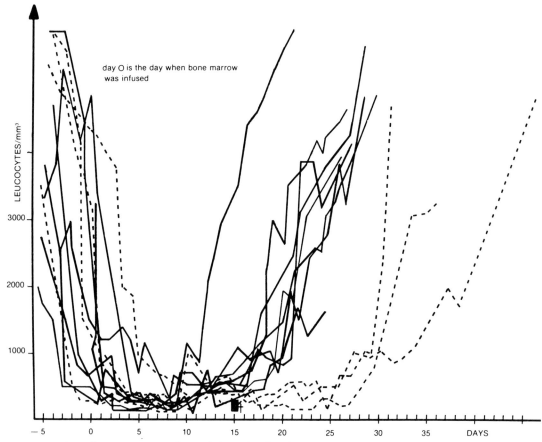

Fig. 2. Recovery of peripheral blood leukocytes in patients treated with high dose combination chemotherapy (TACC) with and without infusion of cryopreserved autologous marrow. — Infusion of autologous marrow. --- No cryopreserved marrow.

Bone marrow aspiration showed recovery of hemopoiesis with some myeloid precursors, a few erythroblasts and immature lymphoid cells between days 5 and 10. Megakaryocytes appeared between days 9 and 15. The kinetics of recovery of peripheral leukocytes were identical in all cases (Fig. 2). Recovery started between day 8 and day 10 (median day 9). Recovery to a WBC count of $1000/mm^3$ occurred between days 13 and 19 (median day 17) (Table 2). The peripheral platelet count reached 50,000 mm^{-3} between days 9 and 28 (median day 15). Reticulocytes (>0.1%) appeared in peripheral blood on days 8-25 (median day 16). There was no relation between the kinetics of recovery and the dose of bone marrow infused.

Patients in Group 1 went into partial remission (50-75% tumor mass reduction), except for the patient with Hodgkin's disease who went into a complete remission. Patients with acute leukemia (Group 2) all went into complete remission and the duration of these remissions, although short (3, 3 and 5 months) paralleled the duration of the first remission phases, during which the bone marrow had been harvested for cryopreservation (3, 6 and 8 months).

In contrast, the high dose combination chemotherapy-induced aplasia seen in Group 3, although not irreversible, appeared to be twice as long as the aplasia in Groups 1 and 2. One patient went into a complete remission (ALL) with a recovery to 1000 WBC/mm^3 on day 30 and a recovery to 50,000 platelets/mm^3 on day 35. This patient, unfortunately, relapsed as early as day 69. Two other patients, unexpectedly resistant to the TACC, slowly recovered a 1000 WBC/mm^3 on days 27 and 28 with 77% and 9% residual circulating leukemic cells. The last patient died on day 15. Post-mortem examination demonstrated severe aplasia with disseminated candidiasis and massive persisting visceral leukemic proliferation.

DISCUSSION

Previous attempts to demonstrate the efficacy of cryopreserved autologous marrow infusion in man to circumvent drug- or radiation-induced myelosuppression, have been unsuccessful either because of spontaneous recovery of hemopoiesis from incomplete myelosuppression (4,22) or because of delayed and partial engraftment (3).

A few trials involving leukemic patients currently in progress seem to indicate autologous engraftment after total body irradiation followed by the infusion of cryopreserved marrow collected during a remission period (9,19). However, except for leukemic patients, total body irradiation has few indications in man, and might be related to a high incidence of non-curable interstitial pneumonitis (14).

The TACC regimen that we used is closely related to the BACT initially designed to condition leukemic patients to allogeneic BMT. It includes CCNU, a long-acting myelosuppressive nitrosourea, which causes a peak of myelo-

TABLE 2. Recovery of peripheral blood cells and tumor response in patients treated with high dose combination chemotherapy (TACC) with and without cryopreserved autologous marrow

Group	Diagnosis	Dose of marrow (10^8/kg)	Storage duration (months)	Leukocytes >1000 mm^{-3} (day)	PMN >500 mm^{-3} (day)	Platelets >50,000 mm^{-3} (day)	Number of platelet transf.*	Reticulocytes >0.1%	Tumor response+
1	NP carcinoma	2.2	1	17	17	15	2	16	PR
1	Rbdmyosarc.	0.8	0.5	12	13	15	5	13	PR
1	Hodgkin's disease	1.9	1.5	18	17	20	5	21	CR
1	Plasmocytoma	0.6	5	16	13	9	1	8	PR
2	AML	0.5	6	17	18	23	8	18	CR
2	A.monoblastic l	1.4	3	19	19	28	9	25	CR
2	A.monoblastic l	0.6	3.5	14	17	14	13**	12	CR
3	ALL	NO INFUSION OF		30	29	33	18	27	CR
3	AML	AUTOLOGOUS MARROW		28 (9% blast cells)	28	no	-	no	Failure
3	CML in acute crisis			27 (77% blast cells)	no	no	-	26	Failure
3	CML in acute crisis			Died on day 15					

*Number of platelet transfusions to maintain the platelet count above 30,000 mm^{-3}. **Patient strongly immunized (anti-HLA +++ 11/12). +CR = complete remission. PR = partial remission.

toxicity 4 weeks after its administration (15). It has been generally assumed in the past that this drug combination, if used alone without bone marrow transplantation, might hopefully result in the eradication of leukemic cells. It would, unfortunately, induce definitive aplasia. Therefore, to the best of our knowledge, such a high dose combination chemotherapy has never been attempted.

In the case of solid tumors, Deisseroth et al. (7) recently used the BACT* regimen with and without cryopreserved marrow in patients with Burkitt's lymphoma. With no marrow infusion, severe granulocytopenia (less than $100/mm^3$) persisted for a median of 19 days and recovery to 500 granulocytes/mm^3 occurred 18-36 days after chemotherapy. In contrast, in autograft recipients, severe granulocytopenia persisted only for a median of 10 days and recovery to 500 granulocytes/mm^3 occurred 14-24 days after chemotherapy. We think that our results bring interesting information concerning the TACC regimen per se and the value of the infusion of cryopreserved autologous marrow. They suggest the following statements: (1) Concerning the TACC regimen, the TACC high dose combination chemotherapy does not induce irreversible aplasia in leukemic patients, nor does it eradicate leukemia. (2) Concerning autologous bone marrow transplantation, combined with high dose combination chemotherapy, the reinfusion of cryopreserved autologous marrow is beneficial in that it shortens the duration of the aplasia by about 50% and it provides a sufficient number of stem cells with normal maturation ability to induce a complete remission in acute leukemia resistant to conventional chemotherapy.

ACKNOWLEDGEMENTS

We are indebted to the nursing staff for the excellent care of the patients; to Mrs. O. Klein and Miss F. Bonnefond for expert technical assistance, and to Miss M. Veillard for typing the manuscript.

REFERENCES

1. Abb, J., Netzel, B., Rodt, H. and Thierfelder, S. (1977): Autologous marrow grafts in dogs given lethal doses of CCNU. Exp. Hemat., 5, Suppl. 2, 43 (Abstract).
2. Ashwood Smith, H.J. (1961): Preservation of mouse bone marrow at -79°C with dimethyl sulfoxide. Nature (Lond.), 190, 1204-1205.
3. Buckner, C.D., Clift, R.A., Fefer, A., Neiman, E.A., Storb, R. and Thomas, E.D. (1974): Treatment of blastic transformation of chronic granulocytic leukemia by high dose Cyclophosphamide, total body irradiation and infusion of cryopreserved autologous marrow. Exp. Hemat., 2, 138-146.

*BACT: BCNU instead of CCNU (TACC).

4. Buckner, C.D., Rudolph, R.H., Fefer, A., Clift, R.A., Epstein, R.B., Funk, D.D., Neiman, P.E., Schlichter, S.J., Storb, R. and Thomas, E.D. (1972): High dose Cyclophosphamide therapy for malignant disease: toxicity, tumor response and the effects of stored autologous marrow. Cancer, 29, 357-365.

5. Buckner, C.D., Storb, R., Dillingham, L.A. and Thomas, E.D. (1970): Low temperature preservation of monkey marrow in dimethyl sulfoxide.

6. Cavins, J.A., Kasakura, S., Thomas, E.D. and Ferrebee, J.W. (1962): Recovery of lethally irradiated dogs following infusion of autologous marrow stored at low temperature in dimethyl sulfoxide. Blood, 20, 730-734.

7. Deisseroth, A., Appelbaum, F., Herzig, G., Graw, R.G., Gorin, N.C., Bull, M., Ziegler, J. and Levine, A. (1977): Bone marrow autografting in a preclinical canine model and in man. In: Abstract Volume, 2nd International Symposium on Immunobiology of Bone Marrow Transplantation, Los Angeles, Calif., June 27-29, 1977.

8. Dicke, K.A., McCredie, K.B., Stevens, E.E., Spitzer, G. and Bottino, J.C. (1977): Autologous bone marrow transplantation in a case of acute adult leukemia. Transplant. Proc., 9, 193-195.

9. Dicke, K.A., Stevens, E.E., Spitzer, G., McCredie, K.B. and Bottino, J. (1977): Autologous marrow transplantation in adult acute leukemia. Exp. Hemat., 5, Suppl. 2, 105 (Abstract).

10. Epstein, R.B., Storb, R., Clift, R.A. and Thomas, E.D. (1969): Autologous bone marrow grafts in dogs treated with lethal doses of Cyclophosphamide. Cancer Res., 29, 1072.

11. Gorin, N.C., Herzig, G., Bull, M.I. and Graw, R.G. (1978): Long term preservation of bone marrow and stem cell pool in dogs. Blood, 51, 257.

12. Gorin, N.C., Stachowiak, J., Hirsch Marie, F., David, R., Muller, J.Y., Jullien, A.M. Cavalier, J., Salmon, Ch., Najman, A. and Duhamel, G. (1977): Greffe de moelle autologue après aplasie thérapeutique définitive entrainant une rémission complète dans un cas de leucémie aiguë myéloblastique chimiorésistante. Nouv. Presse Méd., 6/31, 2741-2745.

13. Graw Jr, R.G., Lohrmann, H.P., Bull, M.I., Decter, J., Herzig, G.P., Bull, J.M., Leventhal, B.G., Yankee, R.A., Herzig, R.H., Krueger, G.R.F., Bleyer, W.A., Buja, L.M., McGinnis, M.H., Alter, H.J., Whang-Peng, J., Gralnick, H.R., Kirkpatrick, C.H. and Henderson, E.S. (1974): Bone marrow transplantation following combination chemotherapy immunosuppression (B.A.C.T.) in patients with acute leukemia. Transplant. Proc., 6, 349-354.

14. Graw, R.G. (1975): Personal communication.

15. Hansen, H.H., Sela Wry, O.S., Muggia, F.M. and Walker, M.D. (1971): Clinical studies with 1,2-chloroethyl-3-cyclohexyl-1-nitrosourea (NSC 79 037). Cancer Res., 31, 223-227.

16. Lewis, J.P. and Trobaugh, F.E. (1964): The assay of the transplantation potential of fresh and stored bone marrow by two in vivo systems. Ann. N.Y. Acad. Sci., 114, 677.

17. Mannick, J.A., Lochte Jr, H.L., Ashley, C.A., Thomas, E.D. and Ferrebee, J.W. (1960): Autografts of bone marrow in dogs after lethal total body irradiation. Blood, 15, 255.

18. O'Grady, L.F. and Lewis, J.P. (1972): The long term preservation of bone marrow. Transfusion (Philad.), 12, 312.

19. Schaeffer, U.W. et al. (1977): Transplantation of fresh allogeneic and cryopreserved autologous bone marrow in acute leukemia. Exp. Hemat., 5, Suppl. 2, 101 (Abstract).
20. Thomas, E.D. and Ferrebee, J.W. (1962): Prolonged storage of marrow and its use in the treatment of radiation injury. Transfusion (Philad.), 2, 115.
21. Thomas, E.D. and Storb, R. (1970): Technique for human marrow grafting. Blood, 36, 507-515.
22. Tobias, J.S., Weiner, R.S., Griffiths, C.T., Richman, C.M., Parker, L.M. and Yankee, R.A. (1977): Cryopreserved autologous marrow infusion following high dose cancer chemotherapy. Europ. J. Cancer, 13, 269-277.
23. Van Putten, L.M. (1966): Monkey and mouse bone marrow preservation and the choice of technique for human application. Bibl. Haemat. (Basel), 11/29, Part 3, 797.

BONE MARROW TRANSPLANTATION (BMT) IN ACUTE LEUKAEMIA WITH
BACT CONDITIONING: RESULTS IN 7 CASES

A. Grañena, C. Rozman, F. Casals, E. Felíu, J. Aranalde,
E. Montserrat and L. Hernández

Postgraduate School of Haematology 'Farreras Valentí', Hospital Clínico y Provincial, University of Barcelona, Spain

SUMMARY

The authors report the results obtained with BACT (BCNU, ARA-C, cyclophosphamide and 6-thioguanine) conditioning and bone marrow transplantation (BMT) in 7 cases of acute leukaemia (4 ALL and 3 AML). Five
attempts of grafting were allogeneic and 2 syngeneic. Three complete
remissions and 2 relatively long survivals (487 days and more than 350
days post grafting) were observed. In 2 cases, the conditioning regimen
has proved to be non-eradicative of the leukaemic process.
    The authors stress the absence of interstitial pneumonia and the
high prevalence of cardiotoxicity in their series. These results are
discussed. A chemotherapeutic strategy in earlier leukaemic phases of
potential candidates for grafting is suggested to reduce the toxicity
and to improve the eradicative efficacy of BACT.

Bone marrow transplantation (BMT) is still an experimental
approach to the treatment of acute leukaemia. Although
usually it has been carried out only in final chemotherapy-
resistant phases of the disease, recently, trials of earlier
grafting in the remission period of leukaemia are in progress (1).
    The results reported in Europe (2) with BMT as treatment
of acute leukaemia have been poor. On the contrary, the
Seattle group have recently presented an encouraging analysis
of their results (1,3,4). Thus, in isogeneic BMT a possible
cure of 30% of patients has been reported (3). Similarly,
these authors observed that in a group of more than 100
acute leukaemia patients the allogeneic BMT produced a
survival plateau of 15% at 2 years. This percentage was
still higher when only patients in good clinical status were
considered (1,4).
    In leukaemia, the conditioning for allogeneic BMT must
fulfill 2 aims: (a) eradication of leukaemia; (b) immunological preparation of the host. For this purpose, the Seattle
group authors have employed a combination of total body irradiation (TBI) and cyclophosphamide (1). The UCLA team has
recommended the association of TBI with a still more aggressive form of chemotherapy (SCARI) (5). Since TBI accounts
for many severe and even fatal complications, chiefly interstitial pneumonia, attempts at conditioning without TBI have

been carried out. With one of such exclusively chemotherapeutic regimens, called BACT, Graw et al. (6) showed that
a long survival can be obtained. However, this type of
conditioning has not been extensively evaluated and further
trials seem justified.

In this paper we report our experience obtained in 7
cases of acute leukaemia treated with BMT and BACT pre-
conditioning

TABLE 1. Patients and type of BMT

Patient No.	Age	Sex	Cytological type of leukaemia (FAB classifica-tion (7))	Type of BMT	Phase of the disease in which the procedure was carried out
1	7	M	ALL (L_2)	Syngeneic	Third relapse resis-tant to chemotherapy; 3 years post diagnosis
2	11	F	ALL (L_2)	Allogeneic	First relapse resis-tant to chemotherapy; 23 months post diag-nosis
3	10	F	ALL (L_2) (Sternberg sarcoma)	Allogeneic	First phase; resistant to chemotherapy 10 months post diagnosis
4	36	M	ALL (L_2)	Allogeneic	First phase; resistant to chemotherapy 7 months post diagnosis
5	24	M	AML (M_1)	Allogeneic	First phase; resistant to chemotherapy 9 months post diagnosis
6	19	F	AML (M_4)	Allogeneic	First relapse, 4 months post diagnosis
7	17	F	AML (M_5)	Syngeneic	BMT as first thera-peutic measure; 1 month post diagnosis

MATERIAL AND METHODS

Table 1 shows the chief characteristics of our patients, the
cytological type of their leukaemia (including the classification according to the FAB cooperative group nomenclature
(7)), the phase of the disease and the type of BMT carried
out. As can be seen, in 1 case (patient No. 7, having a
form of acute monocytic leukaemia), the BMT was implemented
as the first therapeutic measure. In the remaining patients,
the grafting was attempted in the final chemotherapy-resis-
tant phase of the disease.

The 4-day BACT regimen was started 5 days prior to the transplantation according to the following schedule: 7 doses of ARA-C and 7 doses of 6-thioguanine (100 mg/m^2 of each one) were given every 12 hours on days -5, -4, -3 and -2. Four doses of cyclophosphamide (45 mg/m^2/24 hours) were also given on days -5, -4, -3 and -2. Finally, one dose of BCNU (200 mg/m^2) was applied on day -2. In order to prevent uric acid nepropathy and cyclophosphamide cystitis, the conditioning regimen was associated with hyperhydration (4 liters/m^2/24 hours) and electrolyte supplements. Chemotherapy was stopped 36 hours before the bone marrow infusion.

From 5 to 10 days before the bone marrow infusion, all patients were admitted to the isolation unit (reverse barrier with positive pressured and filtered air). At the same time, skin decontamination (bacitracin, neomycin and nystatin) and bowel sterilization (every 6 hours, oral administration of: gentamicin, 200 mg; vancomycin, 500 mg and nystatin 1 x 10^6 μU). Additional support measures included parenteral nutrition, platelet transfusions and granulocyte transfusions.

For the bone marrow aspiration and infusion, the procedure reported by Thomas and Storb (8) was followed strictly. In cases of allogeneic BMT, the prophylactic administration of methotrexate was carried out after the BMT according to the Seattle group schedule (9).

RESULTS

Our results are summarized in Table 2. Two cases (Nos. 5 and 6) out of 7 patients can be considered as good responders to the procedure. In patient No. 5 it was soon evident that the allograft was functioning. Complete remission and complete clinical recovery persisted for 255 days and the survival from the BMT was 487 days. Patient No. 6 developed a severe abdominal infection during the post-grafting period, but evidence of an allograft and complete chimerism could be demonstrated on day 30 post grafting. Complete remission and a good clinical recovery ensued and lasted 275 days. Afterwards, the patient relapsed (from her own original leukaemia) and is still alive (357 days post BMT).

An additional patient (No. 1) achieved a complete remission, but he died on day 30 post grafting due to cardiotoxicity.

The remaining 4 patients died on days 29, 8, 11 and 10 after BMT due to Gram-negative septicaemia. The post-mortem examination showed in 2 cases (Nos. 2 and 4) evidence of persisting leukaemia.

In all our patients some degree of cardiotoxicity was suspected. During BACT conditioning, a pulse rate over 120/min developed in all of them and lasted in the survivors several weeks. EKG showed evidence of sinus tachycardia which could only partially be controlled by administration of digitoxin and/or propranolol. In patient No. 1 the cardiotoxicity was more evident (premature ventricular beats,

TABLE 2. Results of BMT

Patient	Number of marrow nucleated cells infused (x 10^8/kg)	Eradication of leukaemia	Evidence of graft	GVHD	Remission and/or survival post grafting
1	7.5	Yes	Yes; repopulation of bone marrow	No	30 days. Death from cardiotoxicity
2	4.2	No	No	No	20 days. Death from Gram-negative sepsis
3	4	Yes	No	No	8 days. Death from Gram-negative sepsis
4	4.3	No	No	No	11 days. Death from Gram-negative sepsis
5	3.4	Yes	Yes; red cell antigen marker (Jk a !)	No	CR* 255 days. Survival 487 days. Death from relapse
6	2.9	Yes	Yes; sex chromosome markers	Yes clinical Grade I	CR* 273 days. Survival 357 days. Still alive
7	2.03	Yes	No	No	10 days. Death from Gram-negative sepsis

*CR = complete remission.

cardiogenic shock) and fatal. In none of our patients was interstitial pneumonia detected. Finally, in 1 out of 5 allogeneic BMTs, a mild degree of graft-versus-host disease (GVHD) could be detected.

DISCUSSION

As already shown previously (6), the BACT conditioning regimen is an alternative procedure which can produce long-lasting bone marrow grafts and thus it can be suitable for those teams lacking TBI facilities.

An outstanding feature is the complete absence of interstitial pneumonia among our patients. The simplest interpretation of this finding would be to correlate it with the lack of TBI during the pre-conditioning, but other possible explanations should be kept in mind. Thus, it may also be due to the low prevalence of GVHD (a condition which apparently favours the development of interstitial pneumonia (10)) or to the relatively early death of our lost patients.

The subclinical cardiotoxicity associated with BMT for leukaemia seems to be very common (11). However, the frequency of clinical cardiotoxicity appears to be higher in our study than in others. The most likely explanation of this complication is the additive effect due to the use of daunorubicin in the previous phases of the disease. For this reason we avoided the use of this drug in our new programme on BMT for acute leukaemia (12) during the first phase of leukaemic disease of patients who later may become candidates for grafting. In this protocol, each new acute leukaemic patient is immediately screened for an eventual HLA-compatible donor and, if the existence of such a donor is confirmed, the patient receives an induction regimen without daunorubicin and also without other drugs which are components of the BACT conditioning.

In 2 out of 7 patients in our series, the BACT conditioning has proved to be non-eradicative of the leukaemic process. The literature is not quite explicit regarding this point in other series. We try to improve the eradicative efficacy of BACT by avoiding these drugs in the earlier leukaemic phases of potential candidates for grafting. It is possible also that some form of cytoreduction, prior to the BACT conditioning (likewise in the SCARI scheme (5)), might be more eradicative, but obviously the toxic effects would probably increase.

In conclusion, we feel that BACT conditioning and similar chemotherapeutic regimens without TBI deserve further trials in order to define more clearly the place which they may occupy in BMT for leukaemia.

REFERENCES

1. Thomas, E.D., Buckner, C.D., Banaji, M., Clift, R.A., Fefer, A., Fluornoy, N., Goodell, B.W., Hickman, R.O., Lerner, K.G., Neiman, P.E., Sale, G.E., Sanders, J.E., Singer, J., Stevens, M., Storb, R. and Weiden, P.L. (1977): One hundred patients with acute leukemia treated by chemotherapy, total body irradiation and allogeneic marrow transplantation. Blood, 49, 511-533.

2. European Bone Marrow Transplantation Cooperative Group Meeting, Courchevel, March, 1977.

3. Fefer, A., Buckner, C.D., Thomas, E.D., Cheever, M.A., Clift, R.A., Glucksberg, H., Neiman, P.E. and Storb, R. (1977): Cure of hematologic neoplasia with transplantation of marrow from identical twins. New Engl. J. Med., 297, 146-148.

4. Thomas, E.D., Fluornoy, N., Buckner, C.D., Clift, R.A., Fefer, A., Neiman, P.E. and Storb, R. (1977): Cure of leukemia by marrow transplantation. Leukemia Res., 1, 67-70.

5. UCLA Bone Marrow Transplantation Team (1977): Bone marrow transplantation in acute leukaemia. Lancet, 2, 1197-1200.

6. Graw Jr, R.G., Lohrmann, H.P., Buli, M.I., Decter, J., Herzig, G.P., Bull, J.M., Leventhal, B.G., Yankee, R.A., Herzig, R.H., Krueger, G.R.F., Bleyer, W.A., Buja, L.M., McGinniss, M.H., Alter, H.J., Whang-Peng, J., Gralnick, H.R., Kirkpatrick, C.H. and Henderson, E.S. (1974): Bone marrow transplantation following combination chemotherapy immunosuppression (B.A.C.T.) in patients with acute leukemia. Transplant. Proc., 6, 349-354.

7. Bennetti, J.M., Catovsky, D., Daniel, M.T., Flandrin, G., Galton, D.A.G., Gralnick, H.R. and Sultan, C. (1976): French-American-British (FAB) Cooperative Group: Proposal for the classification of the acute leukaemias. Brit. J. Haemat., 33, 451-458.

8. Thomas, E.D. and Storb, R. (1970): Technique for human marrow grafting. Blood, 36, 507-515.

9. Storb, R., Thomas, E.D., Weiden, P.L., Buckner, C.D., Clift, R.A., Fefer, A., Fernando, L.P., Giblett, E.R., Goodell, B.W., Johnson, F.L., Cerner, K.G., Neiman, P.E. and Sanders, J.E. (1976): Aplastic anemia treated by allogeneic bone marrow transplantation: a report of 49 new cases from Seattle. Blood, 48, 817-841.

10. Neiman, P.E., Thomas, E.D., Reeves, W.C., Ray, G.G., Sale, G., Cerner, K.G., Buckner, C.D., Clift, R.A., Storb, R., Weiden, P.L. and Fefer, A. (1976): Opportunistic infections and interstitial pneumonia following marrow transplantation for aplastic anemia and hematologic malignancy. Transplant. Proc., 8, 663-667.

11. Rozman, C. and Estape, J. (1978): Protocolo de tratamiento de los casos de leucemia aguda posibles candidatos a trasplante de medula ósea (existencia de un donante histocompatible) (LATMO$_{E-78}$). In: En Protocolos Oncohematológicos, pp. 35-39. Salvat Ed., Barcelona.

12. Buja, L.M., Ferrans, V.J. and Graw Jr, R.G. (1978): Cardial pathologic findings in patients treated with bone marrow transplantation. Human Path., 7, 17-45.

AUTOLOGOUS BONE MARROW TRANSPLANTATION IN ACUTE LEUKEMIA:
CASE REPORT AND CURRENT PROBLEMS

K.P. Hellriegel, W.D. Hirschmann, Ch. Gauwerky, D. Gerecke,
H. Borberg and R. Gross

Department of Internal Medicine, University of Cologne,
Cologne, Federal Republic of Germany

SUMMARY

Autologous bone marrow transplantation has been performed in a 43-year-
old woman suffering from acute promyelocytic leukemia. The marrow was
harvested during complete remission, cryopreserved and re-infused
during relapse (after thawing, 1.1 x 10^8 mononuclear cells per kg body
weight). For conditioning, a modification of the TRAMPCO scheme was
used. A complete remission lasting 3 months was achieved. Following reappearance of a relapse, chemotherapy for further remission induction
was ineffective, and the patient died on day 155 after autologous bone
marrow transplantation.
    The problems connected with autologous bone marrow transplantation
are discussed: (1) recognition and elimination of residual leukemic
cells in the bone marrow obtained during remission, (2) procedure for
conditioning, and (3) evaluation of the efficacy of autologous bone
marrow transplantation.

In adults with acute non-lymphoblastic leukemia, the rate of
first remissions is now in the range of 50 to 80% (1-5). In
contrast, most cases fail to enter a second remission. Intensive cytostatic therapy may induce bone marrow aplasia,
but repopulation of the marrow with normal hematopoiesis
hardly occurs. Autologous bone marrow transplantation
(AuBMT), the re-infusion of autologous bone marrow obtained
during complete remission, appears to be an alternative for
inducing a second complete remission even in patients with
a poor prognosis following a relapse. The premises for AuBMT
now seem to be fulfilled: highly effective polychemotherapy
and supportive care, cryopreservation, storage and thawing
as well as techniques to measure the viability of hematopoietic precursor cells. The problems and the clinical findings after AuBMT will be demonstrated in a representative
case.

CASE REPORT

In a 43-year-old woman (J.Nr. 08/178-74), acute promyelocytic leukemia was diagnosed in December 1973. Complete remission lasting from April 1974 to April 1976 was achieved by
treatment with three COAP schemes. For remission maintenance,

the patient received 5 further COAP schemes and, during the intervals, 6-mercaptopurine (100 mg/day) and methotrexate (20 mg twice weekly).

In April 1976, a relapse occurred which was complicated by severe disseminated intravascular coagulation (platelets 13,000 per cu.mm; fibrinogen 60 mg/dl, fibrinogen-split products positive, alcohol gelation test positive). The patient was treated with heparin (10 to 15,000 U/day) and a polychemotherapy regimen consisting of 2 mg vincristine and 70 mg doxorubicin on day 1, and 160 mg thioguanine, 12.5 mg methotrexate, and 170 mg cyclophosphamide on days 1 to 5 (Fig. 1). This regimen, a modification of the TRAMPCO scheme (6), was used since the patient was sensitized against cytosine-arabinoside. The same drugs in the same doses were given on days -5, -4 and -3 prior to the transfusion of autologous bone marrow. This marrow was withdrawn and stored in February 1975, 10 months after the patient entered into complete remission and 14 months before the relapse occurred.

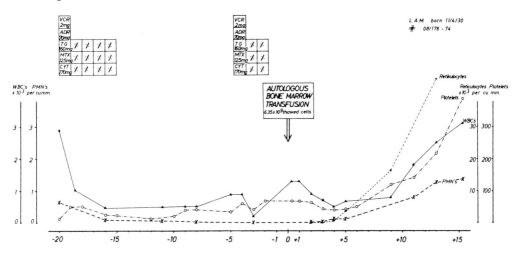

Fig. 1. Conditioning and follow-up of peripheral blood values before and after AuBMT.

Under general anesthesia, 8.5×10^9 cells were obtained by multiple aspirations from the iliac bones under sterile conditions. After the amount of peripheral blood cells was subtracted, 6.8×10^9 bone marrow cells were calculated. The cells were frozen in 2 ml ampoules according to the method described by Schaefer and Dicke (7), the freezing rate was 1° C per minute up to -60° C, and the cells were subsequently stored in liquid nitrogen (-196° C). After thawing, 6.35×10^9 mononuclear cells (recovery of 93%), were counted. Thus, the patient received 1.1×10^8 mononuclear cells per kg body weight. After thawing 9.5 colonies per 10^5 cells were demonstrated by agar colony technique.

At the time of engraftment the bone marrow was aplastic,

as could be shown by biopsy. No adverse reactions were observed, neither during the transfusion phase nor thereafter. During the cytopenic phase the patient received red blood cell and platelet transfusions, if necessary.

Recovery of bone marrow, leukocyte, granulocyte, reticulocyte and platelet counts was disproportionately rapid, and the patient was discharged from hospital in complete remission on day 16 after engraftment. The patient was kept in remission 3 months; for remission maintenance, the cytostatic regimen described was applied twice. In September 1976 a relapse combined with DIC reappeared. Chemotherapy for further remission induction was ineffective. The patient died on day 155 after AuBMT from a candida pneumonia, finally complicated by renal insufficiency.

DISCUSSION AND CONCLUSIONS

In patients suffering from acute leukemia, allogeneic bone marrow transplantation is as yet connected with three main problems: histoincompatibility between donor and recipient, graft-versus-host reaction and recurrence leukemia (8). By using AuBMT it is possible to overcome at least the immunological barriers combined with allogeneic bone marrow transplantation. The disadvantage of this procedure is that the stored and re-infused marrow may still contain viable leukemic cells. The quantity of leukemic cells present in the marrow during remission of acute leukemia is not exactly known. Cytogenetic studies allow differentiation between normal hematopoiesis and the leukemic cell clone in cases having an aneuploid karyotype during relapse. Our own studies demonstrate that about half of the patients with aneuploidy show only diploid mitoses during remission. In the others, however, even during long-term complete remissions (up to 2 years) a percentage of aneuploid metaphases ranging between 2 and 5 can be observed (9). Cytogenetic studies may thus serve as a quality control, as an indicator for the percentage of persisting leukemic cells, which are at least capable of actively dividing and which probably are viable cells. The consequence is that autologous marrow should be harvested when normal hematopoiesis is maximal, and additionally, the percentage of leukemic cells is at its nadir.

Means must be sought to eliminate the residual leukemic cells from the marrow obtained during remission in order to permit re-infusion of autologous marrow containing normal cells only. Haas et al. (10) used a highly absorbed specific anticommon-ALL-globulin which did not alter normal hematopoiesis when added in a concentration necessary for cytotoxic effect. By exposure to heat, drug-resistant leukemic cells may be preferentially eliminated and the risk of a relapse diminished, while the reduction of the number of normal cells seems to be quite acceptable and does not necessarily reduce the frequency of a successful engraftment (11). Another possibility for in vitro separation of normal and leukemic stem cells would be the density gradient technique.

Conditioning of the patients prior to AuBMT strongly depends on the quality of the cryopreserved marrow. After elimination of all leukemic cells, lethal conditioning, as performed for allogeneic bone marrow transplantation, is the best option and provides a reliable means of assessing the success of AuBMT directly. May it, however, be considered justifiable to subject patients receiving autologous bone marrow with still viable leukemic cells to cytostatics plus lethal total body irradiation, merely in order to document the success of a procedure? According to the palliative effect of AuBMT we feel that patients at present should only be conditioned with intensive cytostatic therapy. In not lethally conditioned patients, however, it is more difficult to evaluate the efficacy of AuBMT. In such cases it cannot be excluded with absolute certainty that the recovery of the bone marrow is due to spontaneous regeneration of hematopoiesis. The frequency of second remissions and the time necessary for recovery, however, provide valuable parameters to judge the effectiveness of the procedure, if the group of transplanted patients is compared to a control group treated with the same high-dose chemotherapy regimen. In our case, the rapid and effective hematopoietic recovery, highly unusual in comparable cases, suggests that the application of stored autologous cells had at least a supportive effect on the regeneration of hematopoiesis.

Although AuBMT, so far, has only a palliative effect, storage of autologous bone marrow harvested during complete remission appears to be indicated in most patients with acute leukemia. AuBMT is an alternative therapy in a patient with relapse, in whom allogeneic bone marrow transplantation cannot be performed due to lack of a suitable donor. In those patients for whom a suited donor is available, storage of autologous bone marrow could serve as a security measure, if a severe graft-versus-host reaction or a recurrence of leukemia were to occur after allogeneic bone marrow transplantation.

REFERENCES

1. Bodey, G.P., Coltmen, C.A., Hewlett, G.S. and Freireich, E.J. (1976): Progress in the treatment of adults with acute leukemia. Arch. intern. Med., 136, 1383.
2. Gale, R.P. and Cline, M.G. (1977): High remission-induction rate in acute myeloid leukemia. Lancet, 1, 497.
3. Gerecke, D., Kaulen, H.J., Hirschmann, W.D., Voigtmann, R. and Gross, R. (1975): Erste klinische Erfahrungen mit einem modifizierten COAP-Schema bei akuten Leukosen des Erwachsenen. Verh. dtsch. Ges. inn. Med., 81, 1116.
4. Holland, G.F., Glidewell, O., Ellison, R.R., Wiernick, P., Rai, K., Bekesi, G. and Cuttner, J. (1976): Acute myelocytic leukemia. Arch. intern. Med., 136, 1377.

5. Wiernik, P.H. (1976): Advances in the management of acute non-lymphocytic leukemia. Arch. intern. Med., 136, 1399.

6. Spiers, A.D.S., Costello, Ch., Catovsky, D., Galton, D.A.G. and Goldman, J.M. (1974): Chronic granulocytic leukaemia: multiple-drug chemotherapy for acute transformation. Brit. med. J., 3, 77-80.

7. Schaefer, U. and Dicke, K. (1973): In: Cryopreservation of normal and neoplastic cells. Editors: R.S. Weiner, R.K. Oldham and L. Schwarzenberg. INSERM, Paris.

8. Thomas, E.D., Storb, R., Clift, R.A., Fefer, A., Johnson, F.L., Neiman, P.E., Lerner, K.G., Glucksberg, H. and Buckner, C.D. (1975): Bone-marrow transplantation. New Engl. J. Med., 292, 832--834 and 895-902.

9. Hellriegel, K.P.: Data to be published.

10. Haas, R.J., Netzel, B., Rodt, H., Thiel, E. and Thierfelder, S. (1977): Use of specific antisera against leukemia-associated antigens in diagnosis and treatment of childhood ALL. 6th Meeting ESPHI, Zürich, 1977.

11. Wheldon, T.E. (1976): Exploiting heat sensitivity of leukaemic cells. Lancet, 2, 1363-1364.

III. Immunodeficiency diseases, osteopetrosis

HETEROGENEITY AND PATHOPHYSIOLOGY OF SEVERE COMBINED IMMUNO-
DEFICIENCY DISEASES

Jean-Louis Touraine

Unité INSERM 80, Hôpital E. Herriot, Lyon, France

Severe combined immunodeficiency diseases (SCID) are characterized by the profound impairment of both humoral and
cell-mediated immunities. Despite a relatively homogeneous
clinical appearance, this congenital syndrome has now been
demonstrated to encompass a heterogeneous group of conditions with distinct inheritances, immunobiologic characteristics and molecular abnormalities. The pathophysiology of
SCID is still incompletely understood but different under-
lying disorders in the various forms of the disease suggest
that several pathophysiologic mechanisms - and not only a
stem cell defect - can result in profound alterations of
both T- and B-cell-dependent immunities.

CLINICAL PICTURE

Many patients with SCID present with common clinical characteristics. A family history of already known or suspected
immunodeficiences is frequently found. Typical and severe
infections with a variety of organisms, including Pneumocystis carinii, fungi, viruses, bacteria and parasites, develop
usually after 1 or 2 months of age and lead to death within
the first 2 years of life, if untreated. Sometimes the disorder is inadvertently revealed by a severe complication of
vaccination with live organisms or by a graft-versus-host
reaction following an inappropriate blood transfusion. In
some forms, however, the above-mentioned manifestations may
be associated with other disorders: bone abnormalities
(especially in SCID with deficiency in the adenosine deaminase (ADA) activity (1), dysostosis (short-limbed dwarfism),
amegakaryocytosis, generalized hemopoietic hypoplasia (reticular dysgenesis) or presentation as a Letterer-Siwe syndrome (2). In all forms, an undisputable diagnosis can be
attained easily and rapidly with the presently available
immunologic assays.

PATHOLOGY OF SCID

In every case, a severe hypoplasia of all lymphoid tissues,
including lymph nodes and spleen, is found at autopsy (3).
The pathologic aspects of these hypoplastic lymphoid organs
may, however, vary to some extent with the various forms of

the disease, the degree of infections and a possible graft-versus-host disease.

Various aspects are especially found in the thymus, generally small and mainly consisting of epithelial cells. No cortico-medullary differentiation is observed (3). Hassall's corpuscles are generally absent but they may be found in some cases, especially in SCID with ADA deficiency (1). When thymic biopsies have been performed before severe infections, various types of lesions have been observed (4), confirming some degree of pathology heterogeneity at an early stage of the disease.

GENETIC HETEROGENEITY

Several modes of inheritance of SCID have been documented. There are autosomal recessive forms with ADA deficiency (1), autosomal recessive forms without ADA deficiency (which may still constitute a very heterogeneous group), X-linked forms and sporadic forms. Some of the sporadic forms may be acquired rather than genetic diseases and various viral infections of the fetus have, for instance, been postulated as occasional - and comparatively rare - etiologies of SCID.

IMMUNOLOGIC HETEROGENEITY

Although, by definition, all patients with SCID lack adequate T-cell functions as well as appropriate antibody production, the immunologic findings may be very different from one case to another. With very few exceptions (5), the number of T lymphocytes in peripheral blood is always decreased. This T lymphopenia may, however, be absolute or moderate. In several infants with some T cells at birth, the number of these cells progressively diminished over the first 4 to 6 months. The in vitro proliferative response to phytomitogens is virtually absent. The response to allogeneic cells in mixed leukocyte cultures may be completely absent, reduced, or close to normal (6). Plasma cells are virtually nonexistent but B lymphocytes with surface immunoglobulins (especially IgM and IgD) are often found, sometimes in relatively large numbers (6). Serum immunoglobulins may be lacking or certain classes (IgM) may be found at normal or relatively high concentrations. Some patients with SCID appear to have virtually no marrow T-cell precursors inducible in vitro into HTLA+, E-rosette-forming cells when incubated with thymic factors, while others do have such cells, albeit at low concentration and with a reduced capacity to differentiate under the inductive influence of thymic factors (7). Direct quantitation of thymic factor activity in the serum of such patients demonstrated either reduced or normal thymic secretion (8). The immunologic heterogeneity is, therefore, very pronounced and various associations of the above-mentioned forms have been described. In addition, variations with time, infections and other factors occur. A tendency to a more and more profound

deficiency with a progressive disappearance of any T lymphocyte and any T-cell precursors susceptible to the influence
of thymic factors has been noticed in infants sequentially
studied from birth (7).

PATHOPHYSIOLOGY

With the above-demonstrated heterogeneity of the SCID syndrome, a plurality of causes and pathophysiologies is expected. Some cases of SCID appear to result, as originally
postulated, from a stem-cell deficiency: the reticular
dysgenesis, the SCID associated with other hematopoietic
abnormalities, the SCID without marrow inducible T-cell
precursors and without peripheral T and B lymphocytes may
belong to this group.

In other, more frequent, cases the presence of some B
lymphocytes, of a few T lymphocytes and of a few T-cell precursors argues against a genuine stem cell defect (7). A
blockage of T-cell precursors during very early stages of
T-lymphocyte differentiation would then represent the most
likely cause of many SCID. The variability of certain immunologic findings may reflect the very level of the blockage which seems to be generally related to intrinsic
cellular defects or abnormalities and occasionally may be
associated with extrinsic defects. The spectrum of alterations found in the differentiation of the B-cell system
probably results, then, either from an associated defect at
the level of the B-cell precursors or from the lack of normal T lymphocytes. The latter hypothesis is supported by
the normal development of the patient's B cells and their
progeny when normal T lymphocytes are provided in vitro (9)
or in vivo following a bone marrow (10) or a fetal liver
transplant (11).

Whether the defective thymus development is mostly a
consequence of the lack of colonization by lymphoid cells
or whether it may be the very cause of some SCID cases is
still open for discussion (7, 12-16). A faulty interaction
between thymic epithelial cells and lymphoid precursor cells
could be incriminated in many cases but is this lack of
interaction initially due to an abnormality of T-cell precursors in the majority of cases or may it be sometimes
due to a primary defect of the thymic epithelium? May SCID
occasionally result from a transient abnormality in embryos,
preventing the attraction of stem cells and T-cell precursors to the thymus at the most appropriate time in development (17)?

The identification of the enzymatic (e.g. ADA) deficiencies or other molecular defects resulting in the various
forms of SCID will be of great importance for a more refined
knowledge of the pathophysiologies. The definition of the
levels at which cell differentiation is blocked, as presently performed, is a useful analysis and may help in the
choice of therapies but it does not designate the etiology
nor the real pathophysiology of the diseases. It does not

even specify with certainty at which level of cell differentiation the biochemical abnormality has its initial effects. The discovery of ADA deficiency (1) as a cause of certain SCID has been of great importance and serves as an example for the still unknown causes of other forms. In ADA-deficient patients, the toxic metabolites accumulate in many cells of various tissues. The most susceptible cells appear to be those of the T-cell lineage, the differentiation and proliferation of which are altered. Although the block always concerns early T-cell differentiation, it may appear to occur at slightly different stages of the lymphoid development, depending on the patient and on the evolution phase. The thymic abnormalities are mainly secondary and appear to be reversible during the first months if precursor cells are provided. B cells are less sensitive than T cells to the toxic effects of accumulated metabolites in ADA deficiencies and their further blockage in differentiation may be largely dependent on the lack of T-cell help.

BORDERLINE WITH PARTIAL COMBINED IMMUNODEFICIENCIES, CERTAIN T-CELL DEFICIENCIES AND COMMON VARIABLE IMMUNODEFICIENCIES

There are several diseases which may sometimes be very close to the SCID syndrome. They, however, have distinct characteristics and raise particular pathophysiologic problems. Among the diseases which have been considered by some authors as special variants of SCID, one should mention the Nézelof syndrome or cellular immunodeficiency with immunoglobulins (18), the 'Bare Lymphocyte Syndrome' or combined immunodeficiency with absence of cell-surface HLA-A and -B antigens (19), the combined immunodeficiencies associated with transcobalamin II deficiency (20) or with membrane defects (21). The nucleoside-phosphorylase deficiency is mainly responsible for a T-cell deficiency (22) but, as many other predominantly T-cell deficiencies, some alterations in antibody production may occur.

CONCLUSION

The heterogeneity of the SCID syndrome, suggested on anatomo-clinical and genetic grounds, has been confirmed by recent studies involving analysis of surface markers of lymphocytes, in vitro induction of T- or B-cell differentiation and identification of some molecular defects. Such an heterogeneity should, however, not be misleading: the definition of SCID is precise and its diagnosis readily made. The elucidation of the various pathophysiologic mechanisms will be of basic significance in immunology. It will probably show that, in immunodeficiencies, as in lymphoproliferative disorders, the 'target cell' of the intrinsic or extrinsic initial abnormality often is not the cell whose differentiation is blocked but its ancestor. It will also be of great help in improving the conditions for ante-natal diagnosis and for the treatment of patients with SCID, especially when a compatible donor is not available for a bone marrow transplant and other therapies are considered: transplantation of fetal liver and thymus, transplantation of thymic epithelial cells, enzyme replacement therapies, injection of soluble factors.

REFERENCES

1. Meuwissen, H.J., Pollara, B. and Pickering, R.J. (1975): Combined immunodeficiency disease associated with ADA deficiency. J. Pediat., 86, 169-181.
2. Cederbaum, S.D., Niwayama, G., Stiehm, E.R., Neerhout, R.C., Amman, A.J. and Berman Jr, W. (1974): Combined immunodeficiency presenting as the Letterer-Siwe syndrome. J. Pediat., 85, 446-471.
3. Berry, C.C. (1970): Histopathological findings in the combined immunity deficiency syndrome. J. clin. Path., 23, 193-202.
4. Hong, R.: Personal communication.
5. Buckley, R.H., Gilbertsen, R.B., Schiff, R.I., Ferreira, E., Sanal, S.O. and Waldmann, T.A. (1976): Heterogeneity of lymphocyte subpopulations in severe combined immunodeficiency. J. clin. Invest., 58, 130-136.
6. Seligmann, M., Griscelli, C., Preud'Homme, J.L., Sasportes, M., Herzog, C. and Brouet, J.C. (1974): A variant of severe combined immunodeficiency with normal in vitro response to allogeneic cells and an increase in circulating B lymphocytes persisting several months after successful bone marrow graft. Clin. exp. Immunol., 17, 245-252.
7. Touraine, J.L. (1978): Human T-lymphocyte differentiation in immunodeficiency diseases and after reconstitution by bone marrow or fetal thymus transplantation. Clin. Immunol. Immunopathol., 12.
8. Incefy, G.S., Dardenne, M., Pahwa, S., Grimes, E., Pahwa, R.N., Smithwick, E., O'Reilly, R. and Good, R.A. (1977): Thymic activity in severe combined immunodeficiency diseases. Proc. nat. Acad. Sci. (Wash.), 74, 1250-1253.
9. Seeger, R.C., Robins, R.A., Stevens, R.H., Klein, R.B., Waldmann, D.J., Zeltzer, P.M. and Kessler, S.W. (1976): Severe combined immunodeficiency with B lymphocytes: In vitro correction of defective immunoglobulin production by addition of normal T lymphocytes. Clin. exp. Immunol., 26, 1-10.
10. Griscelli, C., Durandy, A. and Virelizier, J.L. (1979): Selective defect of precursor T cells associated with apparently normal B lymphocytes in severe combined immunodeficiency disease. This volume.
11. Touraine, J.L. (1979): Bone marrow or fetal tissue transplantation in severe combined immunodeficiencies. This volume.
12. Pyke, K.W., Dosch, H.M., Ipp, M.M. and Gelfand, E.W. (1975): Demonstration of an intrathymic defect in a case of severe combined immunodeficiency disease. N. Engl. J. Med., 293, 424-428.
13. Cooper, M.D. (1975): Defective thymus development: A cause of combined immunodeficiency. N. Engl. J. Med., 293, 450-451.
14. Hong, R., Santosham, M., Schulte-Wissermann, H., Horowitz, S.,

Hsu, S.H. and Winkelstein, J.A. (1976): Reconstitution of B- and T-lymphocyte function in severe combined immunodeficiency disease after transplantation with thymic epithelium. Lancet, 2, 1270-1272.

15. Dosch, H.M., Lee, J.W.W., Gelfand, E.W. and Falk, J.A. (1978): Severe combined immunodeficiency disease: A model of T-cell dysfunction. Clin. exp. Immunol., 34, 260-267.

16. Pahwa, R.N., Pahwa, S.G. and Good, R.A. (1978): T-lymphocyte differentiation in severe combined immunodeficiency: Defects of the thymus. Clin. Immunol. Immunopathol., in press.

17. Le Douarin, N.M. and Jotereau, F.V. (1975): Tracing of cells of the avian thymus through embryonic life in interspecific chimeras. J. exp. Med., 142, 17-40.

18. Nezelof, C., Jammet, M.L., Lortholary, P., Labrune, B. and Lamy, M. (1964): L'hypoplasie héréditaire du thymus. Sa place et sa responsabilité dans une observation d'aplasie lymphocytaire normoplasmocytaire et normoglobulinémique du nourrisson. Arch. franc. Pédiat., 21, 897-920.

19. Touraine, J.L., Betuel, H., Souillet, G. and Jeune, M. (1978): Combined immunodeficiency disease associated with absence of cell-surface HLA-A and -B antigens. J. Pediat., 93, 47-51.

20. Hitzig, W.H., Doehmann, U., Pluess, H.J. and Vischer, D. (1974): Hereditary transcobalamin II deficiency: Clinical findings in a new family. J. Pediat., 85, 622-632.

21. Kersey, J.H., Fish, L.A., Cox, S.T. and August, C.S. (1977): Severe combined immunodeficiency with response to calcium ionophone: A possible membrane defect. Clin. Immunol. Immunopathol., 7, 62-68.

22. Giblett, E.R., Amman, A.J., Wara, D.W., Sandman, R. and Diamond, L.K. (1975): Nucleoside-phosphorylase deficiency in a child with severely defective T-cell immunity and normal B-cell immunity. Lancet, 1, 1010-1013.

SELECTIVE DEFECT OF PRECURSOR T CELLS ASSOCIATED WITH APPARENTLY NORMAL B LYMPHOCYTES IN SEVERE COMBINED IMMUNODEFICIENCY DISEASE[x]

C. Griscelli, A. Durandy and J.L. Virelizier

Groupe de Recherches d'Immunologie et de Rhumatologie Pédiatriques, Unité INSERM U 132, Hôpital des Enfants Malades, Paris, France

SUMMARY

Two patients, one with an autosomal and the other a sex-linked form of severe combined immunodeficiency (SCID), had more than 95% B cells in their peripheral blood. Despite an increased absolute number of B lymphocytes, the patients were unable to produce serum antibodies. In each patient, geno- or pheno-identical bone marrow (BM) transplantation was followed by the visualization of a thymus shadow and the appearance of both cellular and humoral functions. Chromosome or allotype studies showed that the T cell originated from the donor while serum immunoglobulins were synthetized by host B cells. In these patients, the pathogenesis appears to be a selective defect of bone marrow precursor T cells without a concomitant intrinsic B cell defect. The successful outcome of the graft in these 2 patients, who are now, respectively, 5 years and 11 months of age and free of infections, indicated that the preferred form of therapy in such cases is a transplantation of bone marrow stem cells which populate the thymus and mature slowly into T cells that cooperate fully with host B cells in synthesis of antibody

It is generally believed that severe combined immunodeficiency (SCID) is due to a defective differentiation of stem cells into T and B cell lines (1). Recently, however, patients have been described whose peripheral B lymphocytes were increased in number but failed to mature into antibody-producing cells (2-6). In this report, we describe 2 unrelated patients in whom bone marrow from HL-A identical donors allowed the development of a thymus that became visible roentgenographically and gave rise to T cells that cooperated with recipient's B cells in the synthesis of immunoglobulin and antibody. In these 2 children the primary defect appears to be a selective abnormality of bone marrow precursor T cells at a prethymic level. The pathogenesis in these patients may therefore be different from that seen in SCID with either an intrinsic defect of stem

[x]This work was supported by INSERM grants (A.T.P. 7-74-28 and 8-74-29) and Fondation pour la Recherche Médical Française.

cells (17), or an apparent intrathymic fault (8,9).

Patient 1. The first patient (S.A.), a girl, was born on 4-24-72 of consanguineous parents who were first cousins. Three of her brothers had died (autopsy performed by Dr. C. Nezelof) before the age of 1, 2 of them from well-documented SCID. The family history suggested an autosomal recessive mode of transmission. The patient was placed in a Trexler isolator (La Calhène, France) 1 week after birth and kept there for 6 months. No attempt was made to decontaminate the child with antibiotic therapy. No lymph nodes were palpable. Tonsils were absent. Routine immunologic studies showed the presence of maternal IgG and trace levels of the other immunoglobulins, but an increased number of B cells and a mild lymphopenia (1000-2600/mm^3) (Tables 1 and 2). Isohemagglutinins were absent and no antibody activity could be detected after immunization with diphtheria and H. pertussis. Delayed skin reactivity could not be demonstrated to DNCB. At day 37 the patient was transplanted with a thymus from a 12-week-old female fetus. In the absence of subsequent clinical and biologic improve-

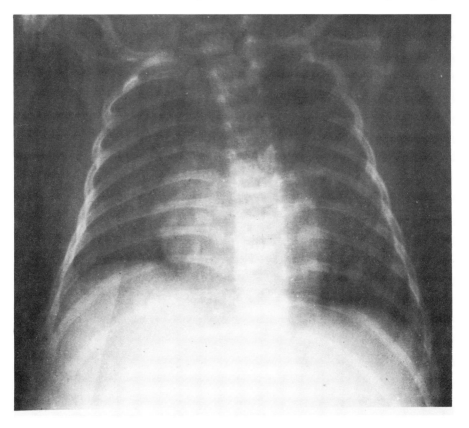

A

118

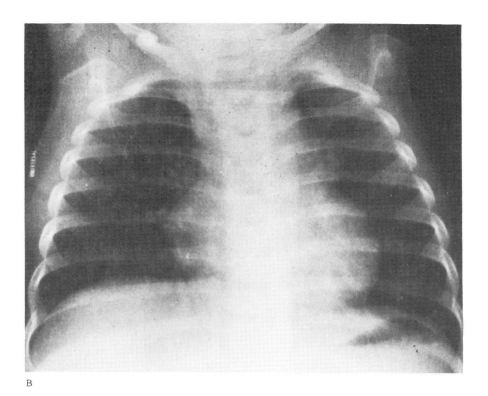

B

Fig. 1. Chest X-rays before (A) and 5 months after (B) bone marrow transplantation (patient 1). A. No thymus visible. B. Thymus normally present.

ment, a transplant of 3 x 10^8 bone marrow cells/kg from an ABO, HLA (A-B-D) histocompatible brother was performed on day 58 (blood group A, HLA: 1-W27/192,12, nonreactive MLR). A mild graft-versus-host (GVH) reaction was observed by day 22 post graft characterized by a transient skin rash and a prolonged neutropenia. A thymic shadow, not previously observed, became apparent 5 months after the marrow graft ((Fig. 1). The patient never received gammaglobulin, and now, at 5 years of age, she has full immunologic reconstitution and enjoys good health.

Patient 2. The second patient (N.G.), a boy, was born on 11-3-1976; the parents were unrelated. Two brothers had died before the age of 8 months from GVH following bone marrow transplantation or blood transfusion. Five maternally related boys had died within the first year of life from infections, progressive vaccinia or BCG sepsis. This family history suggested a sex-linked transmission. In 3 of the 7 patients post mortem examinations (performed by Dr. C. Nezelof) had confirmed the diagnosis of SCID. The patient was placed in a Trexler isolator immediately after a sterile

119

delivery. Forty-two days later, the recovery of 3 different bacteria from the stools prompted decontamination with oral antibiotic therapy for the remaining 6 months of isolation.

No lymph nodes were palpable and tonsils were absent. Routine immunologic studies showed the same findings as that seen in the first patient, i.e., mild lymphopenia (900-3500/mm^3) (Tables 1 and 2), an increase of circulating B cells, the presence of maternal IgG, trace levels of the other immunoglobulin classes, and absence of isohemagglutinins and antibodies after various immunizations. Skin tests to phytohemagglutinin (PHA), and hemocyanin (KLH) remained negative. The patient was transplanted on day 47 with 1.5 x 10^8 bone marrow cells/kg from a maternal aunt who was ABO, HLA (A-B) identical (blood group O, HLA: 1,8/W29,12) but mixed leukocyte reaction (MLR) was slightly positive (cpm/min: 2800, proliferative index: 1.8). Evidence for GVH was obtained 10 days post graft with a recurrent skin rash followed by persistent eosinophilia. A thymic shadow, absent on the first radiographs, became apparent 5 months after the marrow graft. The patient is fully reconstituted, and in good health; he has never received gammaglobulin therapy.

B LYMPHOCYTE FUNCTION (Table 1)

Before transplantation, the B cells of both patients were increased in absolute number (see Table 2). Almost all their lymphocytes (95-100%) carried surface Ig determinants upon labeling with anti-light chains ($\kappa + \lambda$) serum. In the first patient a large percentage of these cells had μ (62%), γ (57%) and α (5%) determinants on their membrane, as previously descrived (10). No attempt was made to identify δ-bearing cells. In the second patient B cells carried μ (60%), δ (97%), γ (43%) and α (1%) determinants. Trypsinization studies, however, revealed that only μ and δ chains were actual products of these cells. A large percentage of these cells carried both μ and δ chains. B cells of this patient also had receptors for complement (83%) and were stained (75%) by a fluorescent anti-serum specific for B cells. At birth, both patients had IgG with maternal Gm type which diminished progressively. Trace levels of IgM (19S) were detectable in both patients but IgA, IgD and IgE were virtually absent. No antibodies appeared following 3 immunizations with pertussis and diphtheria toxoid in the first patient or with tetanus toxoid and purified blood group substances A and B (Benasil-Miami, Fla.) in the second patient. The low levels of antibody to tetanus and pertussis originally seen in the second patient were considered to be of maternal origin and did not increase after subsequent antigenic challenges.

Following transplantation, both patients had a rapid rise in IgM levels by the time of their first signs of GVH reaction. IgM returned to lower levels soon after, but rose progressively together with the 4 other immunoglobulins

	FIRST PATIENT (S.A.)					SECOND PATIENT (N.G.)				
	Before transplant	Days after bone marrow transplant				Before transplant	Days after bone marrow transplant			
		1-30	31-60	91-200	4 years		1-30	31-60	91-200	8 months
IMMUNOGLOBULINS										
IgG (mg/dl)	750*	230	300	780	1800	780*	300	150	184	340
IgM (mg/dl)	<10	87	18	90	220	<10	27	11	14	27
IgA (mg/dl)	< 5	< 5	12	30	120	< 5	< 2	< 2	5	11
IgD (mg/dl)	0	0	0	0	0.1	0	0	0	0	0.01
IgE (U/ml)	<10	<10	<10	<10	200	<10	35	45	80	240
Ig BEARING CELLS (%)										
μ	62	74	61	17	8	60	41	NT	13	6
δ	NT	NT	NT	NT	<1	97	56	NT	19	12
μ + δ	NT	NT	NT	NT	NT	58	NT	NT	12	NT
Light chains (κ + λ)	94	100	83	26	18	95	88	NT	25	NT
ANTIBODY FORMATION**										
Diphtheria (I.U.)	0	0	5	1	NT	NT	1:40	1:40	5	20
Tetanus (I.U.)	NT	0	0	0	0:15	1:30*	1:10	2	31	17
Anti B agglutinins	0	1:4	NT	1:128	1:256	0	1:4	1:8	1:8	1:32
Anti A agglutinins	-	-	-	-	-	0	1:8	1:16	1:16	1:16
H. pertussis	0	0	1:40	1:320	1:10	1:10*	1:80	1:160	NT	1:160
Poliovirus type 1	NT	0	0	1:640	0	0	NT	1:8	NT	1:8
type 2	NT	0	0	1:2560	1:256	0	NT	1:16	NT	1:8
type 3	NT	0	0	1:320	1:16	0	NT	1:8	NT	1:64

*Maternal origin. **The first patient was immunized against diphtheria and pertussis several times before and after transplant. Polioviruses were given shortly after transplantation and tetanus toxoid 2 years later. The second patient was immunized with tetanus toxoid and blood group substances A and B before and after transplant. Pertussis, polio vaccine and diphtheria toxoid were administered after transplantation.

(Table 1). Following new antigenic stimulations, antibodies
to blood group substances and various specific antigens
rose to normal or very high levels. Lymphocytes bearing μ
and δ chains decreased slowly and reached normal values
within 5 months after transplantation. The isohemagglutinins
of the second patient contained a Gm(1+) factor not present
on the immunoglobulins of the donor. Indeed, blood group A
red blood cells (RBC) sensitized with the immune isohemagglutinins present in the serum of the second patient after
immunization with blood group substances were agglutinated
with 2 anti-Gm(1+) antisera.

T CELL FUNCTIONS (Table 2)

Before transplantation, the number of E-RFC was not assessed in the first patient. It was below 1% in the second
child, as was the number of cells reacting with an antiserum specific for T lymphocytes (less than 1% killed in a
cytotoxic test); E-RFC did not increase following incubation of his lymphocytes with a preparation of Thymosin
(fraction V, 50-100 γ/ml for 18 hours) kindly supplied by
Dr. A. Goldstein. Serum thymic factor of this patient was
within normal limits (1:16). In both cases mitogenic proliferation to polyclonal mitogens was absent. The lymphocytes of the first patient responded and stimulated normally in MLR; this has been previously discussed (10).
Fluorescent studies showed that the cells transformed in
the presence of mitomycin-C-treated unrelated lymphocytes,
carried membrane-bound Ig determinants, suggesting that the
B cells of this patient were able to proliferate in MLR.
    After transplantation (Table 2), the number of E-RFC
in the first patient reached normal values 8 months after
transplant. T cells determined by rosetting and anti-HTLA
serum also rose significantly in the second patient and
reached normal values 6 months after transplant. Lymphocytes of both patients rapidly became capable of responding
to polyclonal mitogens. Skin tests also became positive to
various antigens and to PHA. MLR was restored 4 months
after transplant in the 2nd patient.

T AND B CELLS COOPERATIVE STUDIES (Table 3)

In vitro T/B cooperation was not studied in the first patient before grafting. The B cells of the second patient
cocultured with normal T cells in the presence of PWM
matured into cells containing IgM and IgD, but not IgA or
IgG.

CHIMERISM STUDIES (Table 4)

Chimerism was established by identification of grafted
cells. In patients 1 and 2, karyotype studies indicated
that dividing cells in the presence of PHA and PWM were of
donor origin (XY in patient 1, XX in patient 2) when the

122

TABLE 2. Cell-mediated immunity in 2 patients with SCID

	FIRST PATIENT (S.A.)					SECOND PATIENT (N.G.)				
	Before transplant	Days after bone marrow transplant				Before transplant	Days after bone marrow transplant			
		1-30	31-60	91-100	4 years		1-30	31-60	91-100	8 months
LYMPHOCYTES/mm^3	1000-2600	3200-5000	3000-4000	3200	3000	1000-3500	2500	500-2500	500-2000	1200-
E - RFC (%)	NT	NT	8	21	71	< 1	4	9	20	46
SKIN TESTS*										
Candida	Neg.	Neg.	Neg.	+	+	Neg.	Neg.	Neg.	Neg.	Neg.
SK-SD	Neg.	Neg.	Neg.	+	+	Neg.	Neg.	Neg.	Neg.	Neg.
Diphtheria	Neg.	Neg.	Neg.	+	+	Neg.	Neg.	Neg.	+	+
KLH	NT	NT	Neg.	+	NT	Neg.	Neg.	Neg.	Neg.	+
DNCB	Neg.	Neg.	+	+	NT	NT	NT	NT	NT	NT
PHA	NT	NT	NT	NT	+	Neg.	Neg.	Neg.	+	+
IN VITRO RESPONSES**										
PHA	1	15	40	100	83	1	63	33	6	26
PWM	1	15	30	80	42	0	20	8	57	73
CON-A	NT	NT	NT	60	123	0	39	34	17	14
MLR	34.5	NT	NT	23	40	0.5	NT	NT	32	NT

*The second patient who was maintained in sterile condition reacted only to the antigens to which he was sensitized (diphtheria and KHL). **Δ cpm x 10^3.

123

TABLE 3. T/B cooperation in the in vitro maturation of B cells from patient 2 (N.G.) in the presence of normal T cells

Origin of cells		% of cells stimulated		w/PWM for 7 days containing	
T[x]	B	IgM	IgD	IgG	IgA
−	Patient	0	0	0	0
Normal	Normal	77	1	64	35
Normal	Patient[xx]	41	2	2	0
Normal	−	< 1	< 1	1	1

[x]T cells were obtained from the peripheral blood of a normal female by sedimentation of E-RFC. [xx]More than 60% of the cells containing IgM and all the cells containing IgD carried the Y chromosome. All the cells containing IgG and IgA derived from the B cells contaminating the normal T cells.

TABLE 4. Chromosome analysis of patients with SCID and normal male and female controls after bone marrow transplantation

	Cells (%) carrying Y chromosome						
	Quinacrine staining			Karyotype after stimulation by			
	Total lympho-cytes	μ- or δ-bearing cells	Ig-containing cells in PWM stimul. cult.	PHA 3 d.	PWM 3 d.	5 d.	MLR[x] 5 d.
Normal male	85-93	80-92	60-80	100	100	100	100
Normal female	0	0	0	0	0	0	0
Patient 1 (S.A.)	77	3	< 2[xx]	100	100	80[xxx]	86[xxx]
Patient 2 (N.G.)	25	78	70	0	0	NT	NT

[x]Stimulator cells were recognized by a chromosomal translocation. [xx]Out of 120 cells containing IgG, IgM, IgA or IgD, only 2 carried the Y chromosome, suggesting that the majority of these cells were XX cells originating from the recipient. [xxx]The remaining transformed cells (20% and 14% respectively) carried recipient's XX marker. Patient S.A. was grafted with a male and patient N.G. with a female bone marrow.

cultures were terminated at day 3. On the other hand, both donor and recipient cells were detectable in 5-day cultures of lymphocytes from patient 1 that were stimulated with allogeneic cells or PWM. These results suggested that mainly donor T cells were initially stimulated but that recipient

B cells could be subsequently involved in the proliferative process.

Double staining with quinacrine and rhodamin-labeled antisera showed that lymphocytes carrying membrane-bound or intracytoplasmic immunoglobulins did not belong to the donor in the first patient. In the second patient, lymphocytes with surface or intracytoplasmic immunoglobulins were shown to have the recipient's Y chromosome marker.

DISCUSSION

Although several studies now stress the heterogeneity of SCID (11,12), it had been previously accepted that this disease is caused by a defective differentiation of a common precursor into both T and B cell lines (1). Two recent studies, however, have challenged our basic concept of this disease. First, it was demonstrated that bone marrow cells from a patient with SCID could mature into E-RFC and antibody-producing cells when cultured on a monolayer of normal thymus epithelium (8). Second, transplantation of epithelial cells obtained from short-term culture of normal human thymus was shown to reconstitute to varying degrees both humoral and cellular immunity in patients with SCID (9). These studies seemed to indicate that there exists, in some such patients, normal precursors of both lines of cells and that their disease may result from a defect primarily involving the thymus. Although this may be true in certain types of SCID, it can hardly account for all of them. For instance, SCID with severe enzymatic defects (ADA and IP) are generally attributed to an anomaly of stem cell maturation (7,13-15). We now describe 2 patients with SCID with B lymphocytes, in whom the defect was situated at the level of a precursor of the T cell line. Following bone marrow transplantation, an existing thymus gland could be repopulated, becoming visible on radiographs and giving rise to mature T cells. In these patients, the newly arising T cells carried chromosomal markers showing that they originated from donor marrow precursors which presumably matured in the recipient thymus. Although it cannot be completely ruled out that a few T cells contaminating the marrow suspension contributed directly to the restoration of immune functions, it is more probable that the slow rise of mature T cells took place in a functional thymus.

It is generally assumed that following bone marrow transplantation, the grafted precursor cells provide both T and B lineages. T cell chimerism has been amply demonstrated by karyotype studies in several patients who have had marrow transplantation (16-20). Most post-transplant studies using allotype analysis indicate that immunoglobulins are produced by donor cells (18,21-23). In one patient, however, immunoglobulins carrying recipient's Gm markers were found following a marrow transplant (20-24). Allotype studies in our patient No. 2 also demonstrated that the antibodies (isohemagglutinins) produced were of host origin.

In patient No. 1 allotypic differences could not be shown, presumably because the same Gm and Inv types were inherited. Nevertheless, quinacrine staining did establish that the cells bearing and containing immunoglobulins in vitro belonged to the recipient in both patients. Why the donor's B cells, presumably present in the marrow graft, were never identified in the recipient is a matter of speculation. The peripheral monocytes and granulocytes also carried the recipient's markers after reconstitution, only the missing lineage being readily replaced.

In the patients reported here, only the absent T cells needed reconstitution since host B cells proved ultimately capable of cooperating with donor's T cells in antibody production. The appearance of a thymus shadow in both cases as well as the normal level of serum thymic factor in one of them strongly suggest that the thymic epithelium was functional in both patients and that the complete absence of T cell function resulted from a prethymic defect. This situation is different from the Nezelof syndrome (25), which is generally attributed to a primary defect of the thymus gland itself and is characterized by a normal level of immunoglobulins and the presence of a low percentage of T lymphocytes.

The defect in our 2 patients resulted in a syndrome characterized by a virtual absence of T cells and the exclusive presence of B lymphocytes which remained blocked at the level of μ and δ chain expression, perhaps due to the lack of helper cell function. Previous studies of similar patients with SCID had suggested that the humoral deficiency could be secondary to a T cell defect (26,27). This would appear to be the case in our patients. Indeed, in our first patient, they could proliferate with the help of mitomicin-C-inactivated normal cells (one way response in the MLR). In the presence of PWM and normal T cells, the B cells of the second patient were also able to mature into IgM- and IgD-containing cells. Finally, following reconstitution of the T cell compartment by marrow graft, the host B cells became capable of producing normal antibodies to various antigens.

Our observations demonstrate that, in such patients, geno- or pheno-identical bone marrow graft is a good way to achieve a full reconstitution of cellular and humoral functions. Unfortunately, a histocompatible bone marrow donor is not always available. In patients with a prethymic deficiency, the logical alternative seems to be the injection of precursor cells from a fetus. In fact, several fetal liver grafts have been responsible for partial reconstitution of SCID patients (28-30). The recent report stating that various patients with SCID have benefited from injections of cultured epithelium from normal thymus offers a new therapeutic approach, not entailing the risks of GVH reaction (9). It is not yet known whether this procedure will be effective in patients who do not seem to have an intrathymic defect, but one must remember, however, that in most instances of

SCID (including our first patient) transplantation of the whole thymus gland itself did not confer full immune capacities (31-33).

ACKNOWLEDGEMENTS

The authors wish to thank Drs. F.S. Rosen and R. Kauffman for reading the manuscript.

REFERENCES

1. Cooper, M.D., Faulk, W.P., Fudenberg, H.H., Good, R.A., Hitzig, W., Kunkel, H., Rosen, F.S., Seligmann, M., Soothill, J. and Wedgwood, R.J. (1973): Classification of primary immunodeficiencies. N. Engl. J. Med., 288, 966.
2. Seligmann, M., Griscelli, C., Preud'homme, J.L., Sasportes, M., Herzog, C. and Brouet, J.C. (1975): Severe combined immunodeficiency with B lymphocytes and with normal MLC response. In: Birth Defects: Immunodeficiency in Man and Animals, pp. 154-157. Editor: D. Bergsma. Sinauer Associates, Sunderland, Mass.
3. Geha, R.S., Schneeberger, E., Gatien, J., Rosen, F.S. and Merler, E. (1974): Synthesis of an M component by circulating B lymphocytes in severe combined immunodeficiency. N. Engl. J. Med., 28, 726.
4. Preud'homme, J.L., Griscelli, C. and Seligmann, M. (1973): Immunoglobulins on the surface of lymphocytes in fifty patients with primary immunodeficiency diseases. Clin. Immunol. Immunopathol., 1, 241.
5. De Fazio, S.R., Criswell, B.S., Kinzey, S.L., South, M.A. and Montgomery, J.R. (1975): A paraprotein in severe combined immunodeficiency disease detected by immunoelectrophoretic analysis of plasma. Clin. exp. Immunol., 19, 563.
6. Griscelli, C. (1975): T and B markers in immunodeficiencies. In: Birth Defects: Immunodeficiency in Man and Animals, pp. 45-49. Editor: D. Bergsma. Sinauer Associates, Sunderland, Mass.
7. Meuwissen, H.J., Pollara, B. and Pickering, R.J. (1975): Combined immunodeficiency disease associated with adenosine deaminase deficiency. J. Pediat., 86, 169.
8. Pyke, K.W., Dosch, H.M., Ipp, M.M. and Gelfand, E.W. (1975): Demonstration of an intrathymic defect in a case of severe combined immunodeficiency disease. N. Engl. J. Med., 28, 421.
9. Hong, R., Santosham, M., Schulte-Wissermann, H., Horowitz, S., Hsu, S.H. and Winkelstein, J.A. (1976): Reconstitution of B and T lymphocyte function in severe combined immunodeficiency disease after transplantation with thymic epithelium. Lancet, 2, 1270.
10. Seligmann, M., Griscelli, C., Preud'homme, J.L., Sasportes, M., Herzog, C. and Brouet, J.C. (1974): A variant of severe combined immunodeficiency with normal in vitro response to allogeneic cells and an increase in circulating B lymphocytes persisting several months after successful bone marrow graft. Clin. exp. Immunol., 17, 245.
11. Hitzig, W.H., Landolt, R., Müller, G. and Bodmer, P. (1971): Heterogeneity of phenotype expression in a family with Swiss-type agammaglobulinemia: observations of the acquisition of agammaglobulinemia. J. Pediat., 78, 968.

127

12. Rosen, F.S. (1975): Immunodeficiency. In: Immunogenetics and immunodeficiency, pp. 229-257. Editor: B. Benacerraf. MTP, Lancaster.

13. Giblett, E.R., Ammann, A.J., Wara, D.W., Sandman, R. and Diamond, L.K. (1975): Nucleoside phosphorylase deficiency in a child with severely defective T-cell immunity and normal B-cell immunity. Lancet, 2, 1010.

14. Vitendaal, M.P., De Bruyn, C.H.M.M., Oei, J.L., Hosli, P. and Griscelli, C. (1978): A new ultramicrochemical assay for purine nucleoside phosphorylase. Anal. Biochem., 84, 147-153.

15. Virelizier, J.L., Hamet, M., Ballet, J.J. and Griscelli, C. (1978): Impaired defense against vaccinia in a child with T lymphocyte deficiency associated with inosine phosphorylase defect. J. Pediat., 92, 358-362.

16. Gatti, R.A., Allen, H.D., Meuwissen, H.J., Hong, R. and Good, R.A. (1968): Immunological reconstitution of sex-linked lymphopenic immunological deficiency. Lancet, 2, 1366.

17. De Koning, J., Van Bekkum, D.W., Dicke, K.A., Dooren, L.J., Van Rood, J.J. and Radl, J. (1969): Transplantation of bone marrow cells and fetal thymus in an infant with lymphopenic immunological deficiency. Lancet, 1, 1223.

18. Stiehm, E.R., Lawlor, G.J., Kaplan, M.S., Greenwald, H.L., Neerhout, R.C., Sengar, D.P.S. and Terasaki, P.I. (1972): Immunologic reconstitution in severe combined immunodeficiency without bone marrow chromosomal chimerism. N. Engl. J. Med., 286, 797.

19. Yamamura, M., Newton, R.C.F., James, D.C.O., Humble, J.G., Buttler, L.J. and Hobbs, J.R. (1972): Uncomplicated HL-A matched sibling bone marrow graft for combined immune deficiency. Brit. med. J., 2, 265.

20. Vossen, J.M.J.J. (1975): The development of the B immune system in man. Bronder-Offset B.V., Rotterdam.

21. Levey, R.H., Gelfand, E.W., Batchelor, J.R., Klemperer, M.R., Sanderson A.R., Berkel, A.I. and Rosen, F.S. (1971): Bone marrow transplantation in severe combined immunodeficiency syndrome. Lancet, 2, 571.

22. Rubinstein, A., Speck, B. and Jeannet, M. (1971): Successful bone marrow transplantation in a lymphopenic immunologic deficiency syndrome. N. Engl. J. Med., 285, 1399.

23. Yount, W.J., Utsinger, P.D., Gatti, R.A. and Good, R.A. (1974): Immunoglobulin classes, IgG subclasses, Gm genetic markers, and Clq following bone marrow transplantation in X-linked combined immunodeficiency. J. Pediat., 84, 193.

24. Vossen, J.M., De Koning, J., Van Bekkum, D.W., Dicke, K.A., Eysvoogel, V.P., Hijmans, W., Van Loghem, E., Radl, J., Van Rood, J.J., Van der Waay, D. and Dooren, L.J. (1973): Successful treatment of an infant with severe combined immunodeficiency by transplantation of bone marrow cells from an uncle. Clin. exp. Immunol., 13, 9.

25. Nezelof, C., Jammet, M.L., Lortholary, P., Labrune, B. and Lamy, M. (1964): L'hypoplasie héréditaire du thymus: sa place et sa responsabilité dans une observation d'aplasie lymphocytaire normoplasmocytaire et normoglobulinémique du nourrisson. Arch. franç. Pédiat., 21, 897.

26. Geha, R.S. (1976): Is the B-cell abnormality secondary to T-cell abnormality in severe combined immunodeficiency? Clin. Immunol. Immunopathol., 6, 102.

27. Seeger, R.C., Robins, R.A., Stevens, R.H., Klein, R.B., Waldmann, D.J., Zeltzer, P.M. and Kessler, S.W. (1976): Severe combined immunodeficiency with B lymphocytes: in vitro correction of defective immunoglobulin production by addition of normal T lymphocytes. Clin. exp. Immunol., 26, 1.

28. Keightley, R.G., Lawton, A.R. and Cooper, M.D. (1975): Successful fetal liver transplantation in a child with severe combined immunodeficiency. Lancet, 2, 850.

29. Ackeret, C., Plüss, H.J. and Hitzig, W.H. (1976): Hereditary severe combined immunodeficiency and adenosine deaminase deficiency. Pediat. Res., 10, 67.

30. Buckley, R.H., Whismant, J.K., Schiff, R.I., Gilbertsen, R.B., Huang, A.T. and Platt, M.S. (1976): Correction of severe combined immunodeficiency by fetal liver cells. N. Engl. J. Med., 294, 1076.

31. Rachelefsky, G.S., Stiehm, E.R., Amman, A.J., Cederbaum, S.D., Opelz, G. and Terasaki, P.I. (1975): T-cell reconstitution by thymus transplantation and transfer factor in severe combined immunodeficiency. Pediatrics, 55, 114.

32. Amman, A.J., Wara, D.W., Salmon, S. and Perkins, H. (1973): Thymus transplantation. Permanent reconstitution of cellular immunity in a patient with sex-linked combined immunodeficiency. New Engl. J. Med., 5, 5.

33. Griscelli, C., Durandy, A., Ballet, J.J., Prieur, A.M. and Hors, J. (1977): T and B cells chimerism in two patients with severe combined immunodeficiency (SCID) after transplantation. Transplant. Proc., 9, 171.

CORRECTION OF SEVERE COMBINED IMMUNODEFICIENCY BY FETAL
LIVER TRANSPLANT. REPORT ON 2 PATIENTS[*]

M. Fiorilli[1], P. Ammirati[1], R. Paganelli[1] and F. Aiuti[2]

[1]Department of Internal Medicine III, and [2]Department of
Infectious Diseases, University of Rome, Italy

It is now possible to distinguish a severe combined immunodeficiency (SCID) characterized by the absence of T and B
cells (1) from SCID having a normal complement of B cells;
this is presumably due to a defect of pre-T cells (2). In
addition, bone marrow cells of other SCID patients can
transform into mature T and B cells after incubation in
vitro or treatment in vivo with thymic epithelium or thymic
hormones (3,4). The fault is probably secondary to the
thymus development. In patients with SCID, bone marrow transplantation (BMT) remains the best treatment whenever histocompatible donors are available.

However, the majority of these patients will not have
compatible donors, and in the past 3 years alternative
therapy with fetal cells has been attempted with some success in a few centers (5,6,7). Previous transplanted cases
reported transient or chronic graft-versus-host reaction
(GVHR) graded from severe to mild. The present report de-
scribes the fetal liver transplant results in 2 SCID patients. Reconstitution of immunological function was
achieved, but a GVHR developed and this was especially
severe in one child.

CASE REPORTS AND RESULTS

Patient 1, S.T., a 2-month-old male, was admitted to the
hospital with interstitial pneumonia and a history of diarrhea, weight loss, and oral moniliasis since the first
month of life. One brother had died from infection in early
infancy. Lymph nodes were not palpable. X-rays revealed an
absence of thymic shadow and typical image of interstitial
pneumonia. Routine immunological studies showed the presence
of maternal IgG and anti-A and B agglutinins, but an absence of serum IgM (for the methodology see our previous
papers Nos. 7 and 8). Bone marrow biopsy confirmed the absence of plasma cells. B and T cells were absent in peripheral blood. The level of adenosine deaminase (ADA), nucleoside-phosphorylase (NP) and thymic hormone were within

[*]Supported by a grant from the National Council of Research of Italy
for Immune Defects, 1977-1978.

normal ranges before and after transplant. Because the health of the patient worsened in the 3rd and 4th month, and a potential donor for BMT was not available, we decided to perform a fetal liver transplant. The patient was transfused with 60×10^6 mononucleated liver cells obtained from a non-living embryo 7 to 8 weeks of age. The patient did not improve clinically during the first 2 months. In the third month, a mild GVHR developed and was characterized by morbilliform, maculopapular skin rash, diarrhea and increase in eosinophil counts. The rash was followed by exfoliation for 2 to 3 weeks. The child's weight did not increase until the first year. After 6 months from transplant there was clinical improvement, regression of pneumonia and oral candidiasis. Eighteen months later the patient was asymptomatic, his weight increased and the immunological responses recovered (Table 1). However, IgA was undetectable in the serum.

Patient 2, F.S., a boy, was immediately admitted to the department of pediatrics of Florence after birth because family history suggested a SCID. In fact, 3 maternal uncles and a brother had died from infection in early infancy. The brother's death was probably complicated by a GVHR which occurred after a blood transfusion. That T cells were absent was tested by the E-rosette technique and by using anti-T serum. In addition, there was an absence of mitogenic response to PHA, Con-A and mixed leukocyte culture (MLC), negative skin tests and absence of serum IgA and IgM. The percentage of surface membrane immunoglobulin (sm Ig) binding cells was normal; the level of ADA was 1.24 mg%/ml of lysate; the NP 38.7 mU/mg; thymic hormone 109.6 πM, all these data were normal. Thymic shadow at Rx examination was present. All these data remained unvaried in repeated controls until the age of 3 months, when the infant presented severe diarrhea and oral moniliasis. He failed to thrive and developed physical signs of pneumonia. The patient was transferred to our hospital for immunotherapy (April 1977). Chest X-rays showed an interstitial pneumonia, which suggested a pneumocystis carinii infection. Because the patient was affected by a SCID with normal B cells and an absence of T cells, we treated him with thymosin (1 mg/kg/day) for 1 week without clinical or immunological benefit. An HLA-compatible bone marrow donor was not available and for these reasons we injected intravenously 50×10^6 nucleated liver cells of a 7-week-old human embryo. After 1 month the infant developed a generalized maculopapular rash, fever, diarrhea and partial alopecia. After 3-4 weeks he showed generalized desquamation of the skin. At the same time there was an increase of eosinophils to 50-70%; skin biopsy showed vacuolization, hyperkeratosis and spongiosis of the epidermal basal layer. No treatment was instituted for the first 6 months. The rash regressed partially. Repeated determination of liver enzymes and other laboratory tests were normal. After 4 months the eosinophil number decreased (<10%) but diarrhea

TABLE 1. Humoral and cellular immunity in patient No. 1 before and after transplant

	Before	Months after transplant						
		2	4	6	8	12	16	18
Lymphocytes/mm^3	600-900	750	500	3100	3000	3450	2000	3040
Serum IgG/mg/ml[*]	780-330[*]	120	80	370	530	590	880	1340
Serum IgM	12-0	0	5	64	82	240	174	140
Sm Ig b. cells IgM[**]	0	0	2	4	11	16	12	11
cells IgD	0	0	1	2	5	6	ND	5
Anti-AB agglutinins	80[*]	0	0	0	8	8	16	32
Anti-O strept.	330[*]	50	0	0	0	125	330	330
E-rosettes (%)	0-3	0	15	45	53	50	58	55
PHA response[***]	2000	2750	78000	53000	55000	45000	50000	42000
Con-A	1500	ND	40000	30000	34000	15000	20000	22000
SPA (staphylococcus)	500	ND	13000	ND	15000	18000	12000	20000
Skin test SK-SD[****]	neg	ND	neg	ND	neg	+	++	++
Candida	neg	ND	neg	ND	neg	+	+	++

[*]Maternal origin. IgA was never detected in serum. [**]Surface membrane binding lymphocytes in %.
[***]The mitogenic response is expressed in c.p.m./min, mean values of 3 samples. Normal values of
10^5 cells expressed in c.p.m.: PHA (34000-80000), Con-A (25000-65000), SPA (10000-22000).
[****]SK-SD streptokinase-streptodornase antigens.

and failure to thrive persisted. However, the general clinical condition improved as well as the oral moniliasis and the pneumonia. Normalization of erythrocyte-sheep red blood cells (E-SRBC) occurred while the B cells decreased in percentage after 2 months and then persisted within the normal values for 1 year. The ratio between T and B was also normal (41% and 20% respectively). Mitogenic response to PHA, Con-A and Staphylococcus protein A (SPA) was normal for a period of 6 months, while in the last month a diminution of PHA response was observed. The lymphocyte reactivity in the MLC test was always below normal values. The HLA typing performed several times before and after transplant was the following: father HLA-A 10, A 11, 4a, 4b; mother HLA-A 1, A 9, B W35. Patient before: HLA-A 10, A 9, B W35, 4a, 4b; 3 months after transplant HLA-A 9, A 2, B 35, B 5, and 1 year and 7 months later unvaried. The HLA typing was performed with similar results on pure fractionated T and B cells after transplantation. However, after 14 months the HLA typing was A 2, A 9, A 10, B 5, BW 35, 4a, 4b. Serum IgM began rising 3 months after transplant and was 500 mg/100 ml for 3.4 months and then decreased to within the normal range in the first year after transplant. Serum IgG was synthesized only during the last 3 months of observation and was homogeneous. IgA was detected only after one plasma infusion.

DISCUSSION

Recent successes in conferring immunological competence on infants with SCID by infusion of fetal liver cells (5,6,9, 10) together with our present report confirm the usefulness of this approach as an alternative form of therapy. In the last 3 years approximately 10 infants with SCID were reconstituted with a survival of more than 6 months.

In some SCID variants with associated thymic aplasia, the combined use of fetal thymus and liver provided immunological reconstitution (11). Our 2 patients with SCID were basically different, since 1 showed an absence of T and B cells, while the second had normal B cells. In the latter patient there was probably only a pre-thymic cell defect, and the absence of plasma cells and antibodies was secondary to a lack of helper T cells. The first patient had an uncomplicated course after transplant, since immunological reconstitution occurred after 3 months and was accompanied by regression of infections, weak and transitory GVHR. However, after 18 months, weight is still below normal. Probably in this patient the transfused fetal liver cells were responsible for immunological reconstitution of both B and T cells, as demonstrated by chromosome markers. 50% of patients with SCID showed a reconstitution of T cells after liver transplant only.

The severe GVHR in patient 2, documented by skin biopsy, chronic diarrhea, increase in eosinophil counts, is an interesting and unusual finding. Severe GVHR is not a frequent complication of fetal liver transplants. In fact, it has occurred and has been fatal only in 1 out of 10 transplanted patients, according to the literature (6). In addition, none of the 5 transplanted SCID patients reported by O'Reilly developed severe GVHR (personal communication). Probably the use of germ-free isolation and/or sterilization of the gut and subsequent recolonization with non-pathogenic flora can play an important role. The protein-losing entheropathy seen in patient 2 can also be secondary to GVHR involving the mesenteric nodes and intestinal mucosa. We can exclude nutritional deficiencies and zinc deficiency since appropriate therapy with medium chain triglycerides and zinc was unsuccessful in patient No.2. We did not administer immunosuppressive drugs for GVHR because the syndrome was not constantly present and we wished to avoid other infections. Since extra-HLA antigens were not present before transplant in patient No. 2, and 2 antigens on total lymphocytes and on fractionated T and B cells appeared, we can assume that these antigens were derived from donor cells.

In conclusion, despite the severe GVHR manifested in 1 patient, we believe that the use of fetal liver is of therapeutic value as an alternative to non-compatible BMT.

REFERENCES

1. Good, R.A. (1978): In: Immunodeficiency. Edited by the Japan Medical Research Foundation. University of Tokyo Press.
2. Seligmann, M., Griscelli, C., Preud'homme, J.L., Sasportes, M., Herzog, C. and Broute, J.H. (1974): Clin. exp. Immunol., 17, 245.
3. Pyke, K.W., Dosch, H.M., Ipp, M.M. and Gelfand, E.W. (1975): New Engl. J. Med., 28, 421.
4. Hong, R., Santhosam, M., Schultze, H., Horowitz, S., Hsu, S.H. and Winkelstein, J.A. (1976): Lancet, 2, 1270.
5. Keightly, R.G., Lawton, A.R. and Cooper, M.D. (1975): Lancet, 2, 850.
6. Buckley, R.H., Whisnant, J.K., Schiff, R.I., Gilbersten, R.B., Huang, A.T. and Platt, M.S. (1976): New Engl. J. Med., 294, 1076.
7. Aiuti, F., Cerottini, Coombs, R.R.A. et al. (1974): Scand. J. Immunol.
8. Aiuti, F., Businco, L., Griscelli, C., Touraine, J.L. and Webster, A.L. (1977): Z. Immun.-Forsch., 153, 95.
9. Rieger, C.H., Lustig, J.V., Hirschorn, R. and Rothberg, R.M. (1977): J. Pediat., 90, 707.
10. Griscelli, C., Durandy, A., Virelizier, J.L., Ballet, J.J. and Daguillard, F. (1978): Pediatrics.
11. Pahwa, R., Pahwa, S., Good, R.A., Incefy, G. and O'Reilly, R. (1977): Proc. nat. Acad. Sci. (Wash.), 74, 3002.

BONE MARROW OR FETAL TISSUE TRANSPLANTATION IN SEVERE COM-
BINED IMMUNODEFICIENCIES

Jean-Louis Touraine
on behalf of the Lyon & St Etienne Bone Marrow Transplant
Team
(with the collaboration of B. Bétend, H. Bétuel, B. Chataing,
L. Cret, R. François, F. Freycon, C. Genin, R. Gilly, M.
Jeune, F. Larbre, B. Lauras, P. Monnet, N. Philippe, H.
Plauchu, B. Salle, G. Souillet, F. Touraine and
A. Valancogne)

Unité INSERM 80, Hôpital E. Herriot, Lyon, France

Eight patients with severe combined immunodeficiency diseases (SCID) were treated and sequentially investigated in
Lyon and St Etienne: 4 infants received a bone marrow transplant (BMT) from an HLA identical sibling; the other 4 were
lacking a compatible bone marrow donor and were thus transplanted with fetal liver and thymus combined.

SEVERE COMBINED IMMUNODEFICIENCY DISEASES

The 8 patients reported had very typical, though varied,
forms of SCID. They all had lymphopenia and decreased percentages of T cells with surface differentiation antigens
(HTLA[+]) and forming E rosettes. No in vitro proliferative
response to PHA or Con A could be demonstrated and the allogeneic response was weak or absent. The numbers of immuno-
globulin-bearing B cells were variable but there were no
plasma cells and virtually no identifiable antibody synthesis in any of the patients although serum IgM levels were
relatively high in some of them. Two patients had a genetic
deficiency in adenosine deaminase (ADA) activity, the others
did not. In the induction assay, involving differentiation
of marrow T-cell precursors into HTLA[+] cells or E-rosette
forming cells, under the influence of thymic factors (1),
all patients proved to have either no or a significantly
reduced number of inducible T-cell precursors (2).

BONE MARROW TRANSPLANTS

Each of the 4 infants treated with bone marrow transplantation had a HLA A, B and D identical sibling. Donor and recipient were of the opposite sex in 3 cases (Table 1). ABO
incompatibility was present in 1 instance. Bone marrow
transplantation consisted in the intravenous infusion of
1.5×10^8 marrow nucleated cells per kg body weight (3). As
shown in the Table, 3 of the 4 patients were immunologically
reconstituted and are now alive, in a perfect condition, 3

TABLE 1. Bone marrow and fetal liver transplantation in SCID

Patient	Treatment	Take	GvHR	Reconstitution	Outcome	Follow-up
*T. ♂	BMT (sister)	+	+	Full	Perfect	> 3 years
C. ♀	BMT (sister)	+	−	Almost full	Perfect	> 3 years
M. ♂	BMT (sister)	+	−	Full	Perfect	> 3 years
H. ♀	BMT (brother)	+	−	Beginning only	Died of previous BCG infection	1 month
S. ♂	FLTT	+	−	Almost full	Perfect	18 months
*B. ♂	FLTT	?	−	No	Died of previous BCG infection	1 month
C. ♀	CETT+FLTT	?	−	Initial ?	Satisfactory in sterile isolation	3 months
F. ♀	FLTT	?	−	Initial ?	Satisfactory in sterile isolation	1 month

BMT : bone marrow transplant(s)
FLTT : fetal liver and thymus transplant(s)

CETT : cultured epithelial thymus transplants
* Patients with ADA deficiency

to 4 years later. Following the transplants, evidence of engraftment (XX chromosomes in male recipients, Gm immunoglobulin groups) was obtained. A mild to moderate graft-versus-host reaction (GvHR) developed in the first patient only and it spontaneously disappeared. In patients T., C. and H., a second marrow transplant from the same donor was performed. No GvHR occurred following the second transplant. The number of peripheral blood lymphocytes increased. Inducible T-cell precursors were found in virtually normal concentration in bone marrow and blood 1½ months after transplantation. Sequential T-lymphocyte differentiation was demonstrable (2). B lymphocytes gave rise to their progeny, the immunoglobulin-secreting plasma cells. The infant with an ADA deficiency exhibited an increased ADA activity in blood lymphocytes. The fourth patient (H.) presented with a severe and generalized BCG infection, the evolution of which was not interrupted by the marrow transplants.

FETAL LIVER AND THYMUS TRANSPLANTS

Fetal liver and thymus transplants (FLTT) consisted in the intraperitoneal injection of all liver and thymus cells obtained from an 8-10 week old fetus. Among the 4 patients treated with FLTT, one has been followed 1½ years (Table). This infant received 2 FLTT and has now a virtually complete immunological reconstitution. T lymphocytes developed from the second donor's precursor cells and they express 4 HLA specificities different from those of the patient's own cells. These T lymphocytes slowly proliferated and matured along the same differentiation pathways as described following bone marrow transplantation (2). More than 6 months were, however, required before a very substantial increase in HTLA[+], E-rosette forming cells was found in the peripheral blood. Weeks later the responses to allogeneic cells and to phytomitogens developed. B Lymphocytes exhibit HLA antigens of the recipient but now appear capable of maturation. Antibody production has recently been demonstrated in this child, following administration of several antigens. Since the patient has been taken off isolation, he developed a few minor infections, readily cured, and he was capable of limiting the virus spread in spite of completely different HLA haplotypes between T lymphocytes and infected target cells. He is presently in perfect condition without further therapy. Such results demonstratively confirmed the in vivo sequence of T lymphocyte differentiation following transplantation of even more immature cells than bone marrow cells. They also suggest that some degree of T-cell B-cell cooperation and some degree of T-cell cytotoxicity may be possible in the face of HLA incompatibility. It, however, remains to be determined whether lymphoid precursor cells maturated in the contact of the recipient's or the donor's thymic epithelial cells. The precise varieties of antibody synthetized, the cytotoxic activity of T lymphocytes on various well-defined target cells and the long-term clinical efficacy also need further investigation.

Another infant had a generalized BCG infection prior to FLTT and died of this infection despite the transplants and antibiotics. The last 2 SCID patients are presently in good condition but they have been treated too recently to allow any conclusion as regards immunological reconstitution. One of these infants had previously received 2 transplants of cultured epithelial thymic cells without significant improvement.

On the whole, experience with treatment of SCID in Lyon and St Etienne confirms the remarkable efficacy of bone marrow transplants from compatible donors and suggests that combined fetal liver and thymus transplants (4) may be of value when no compatible bone marrow donor is available.

REFERENCES

1. Touraine, J.L., Incefy, G.S., Touraine, F., Rho, Y.M. and Good, R.A. (1974): Differentiation of human bone marrow cells into T lymphocytes by in vitro incubation with thymic extracts. Clin. exp. Immunol., 17, 151-158.
2. Touraine, J.L. (1978): Human T-lymphocyte differentiation in immunodeficiency diseases after reconstitution by bone marrow or fetal thymus transplantation. Clin. Immunol. Immunopathol., 12, in press.
3. Touraine, J.L., Freycon, F., Chataing, B., Souillet, G., Salle, B., Philippe, N., Betuel, H., Lauras, B., Touraine, F., Jeune, M. and Monnet, P. (1978): Experience with bone marrow transplantation for severe combined immunodeficiencies in Lyon and Saint-Etienne. Pathologie-Biologie, 26, 27-28.
4. Pahwa, R., Pahwa, S., Good, R.A., Incefy, G.S. and O'Reilly, R.J.

(1977): Rationale for combined use of fetal liver and thymus for immunological reconstitution in patients with variants of severe combined immunodeficiency. Proc. nat. Acad. Sci. (Wash.), 74, 3002-3005.

LYMPHOID CELL TRANSPLANTATION IN EXPERIMENTAL AND HUMAN OSTEOPETROSIS

Jean Jacques Ballet[1], René Moutier[2], Claude Griscelli[3] and Kyoko Toyama

[1]Unité INSERM U-108, Hôpital Saint-Louis, Paris, [2]Centre de Sélection et d'Elevage des Animaux de Laboratoire, CNRS, and [3]Unité d'Immunohématologie, Hôpital des Enfants-Malades, Paris, France

Osteopetrosis is a condition defined by a generalized increased density of bones due to severe impairment of bone resorption (1). In studies on osteopetrotic mutant rodents, the decisive observation was the obtaining of a cure by temporary parabiosis (2). Demonstration of cell mediation was obtained using cell transplantations, which induced a reversal (3,4) as well as an induction of osteopetrosis in mice (5).

In rats, 3 independent (6) mutations are known: (1) the 'ia' mutant, with temporary osteopetrosis (7) and abnormal osteoclast functions (8); (2) the 'tl' mutant, in which no resorption was observed after cell transplantation (9); and (3) the 'op' mutant (10), in which parabiosis (11) and bone marrow transplantations (12,13,14) were effective.

Human osteopetrosis (cf. 15), in its progressive form, inherited as if determined by an autosomal recessive gene, is usually revealed early in life with severe hematological symptoms, optic atrophy, and other symptoms related to an abnormal bone resorption (16). Another form, with milder manifestations, is usually discovered later in life.

Four infants with severe osteopetrosis were transplanted with bone marrow or fetal lymphoid cells (17,18,19, 20). Taking into account the risks of an immunosuppression in a situation where mechanisms and immunological status were not entirely defined, these first attempts in man were performed by injecting cells from related donors or fetuses without any immunosuppressive preparation.

Pertinent clinical, biological and immunological data are given in Tables 1 and 2. Transplantation data are indicated in Table 3. In 2 cases (Nos. 3 and 4), no improvement was observed in blood pictures or bone X-rays. Despite blood transfusions and steroid therapy, the clinical evolution is unfavorable more than 1 year after transplantation.

In case No. 2 a temporary hematological improvement was observed at day +30 after transplantation. By day +60 metaphyseal resorption was visible, with a slight resorption in some long bones, but by day 120 a generalized bone densification had reappeared, and immature cell numbers in peripheral blood were again increasing.

TABLE 1. Clinical and biological data (at the dates of cell transplantation)

Case No.	1	2	3	4	
Sex	Female	Male	Female	Female	
Age (months/days)	2/26	1/25	6/7	7/19	9/16
Size (cm)	52	60	63	64	N.A.
Spleen/Liver enlargement	+ + +	+	+ + +	+ + +	+ + +
Optic atrophy	+ +	0	+	+ +	+ +
Hemoglobin (g/100 ml)[x]	9.6	7.4	9.9	6.7	9.2
Immature nucleated cells in peripheral blood	+ +	+ + +	+ +	0	+
Reticulocytes (per mm^3)	170000	310000	512000	336000	180000
Thrombocytes (per mm^3)	20000	65000	35000	10000	30000

[x]All patients, except case No. 2, had received prior blood transfusions.

TABLE 2. Immunological data (at the date of first cell transplantation)

Case No.	1	2	3	4
Age	2/26	1/25	6/7	7/19
IgG (serum, mg/100 ml)	850	320	1050	650
IgM (serum, mg/100 ml)	64	62	210	110
IgA (serum, mg/100 ml)	60	38	90	56
Allohemagglutinins (serum)	Detectable	Undetectable		High
Antibody function (serum)	-	±	+	+
Lymphocytes (blood)				
Absolute number (per mm^3)	2500-5000	5000-15000	6000-8000	6000-20000
E-rosetting lymphocytes[x] (%)	35	24	7	24
μ-bearing lymphocytes[x] (%)	N.D.	N.D.	14	8
In vitro proliferative response of blood lymphocytes to:[xx]				
Lectins (phytohemagglutinin, pokeweed mitogen, concanavalin-A)	Normal	Normal	Normal	Normal
Mixed leukocyte reaction[xx]	Positive	Positive	N.D.	Positive
Skin test (phytohemagglutinin)	Positive	N.D.	N.D.	N.D.

[x]Lymphocytes sedimenting on a Ficoll Hypaque gradient. [xx]Lymphocytes sedimenting in layers 25% to 35% on bovine serum albumin, response to lymphocytes from an unrelated donor.

TABLE 3. Transplantation data

Case	1	2	3	4
Sex (recipient)	Female	Male	Female	Female
HL-A (A, B) types (recipient)	A2,W17/192,B14	A9,A1/BW25,B8	A3,-/W29,12	A3,B7/A28/B12
Donor and injected cells	Sister (bone marrow, i.v.)	Unrelated fetus (liver, i.p., thymus, i.v.)	Father (bone marrow, i.v.)	1) Father (bone marrow, i.v.) (twice) 2) unrelated fetuses (thymus, i.v.)
Number of injected nucleated cells (per kg weight)	0.7×10^9	Liver : 1.87×10^8 Thymus: 4.5×10^5	6.3×10^9	1) 0.08 and 1.6×10^9 2) 19×10^6

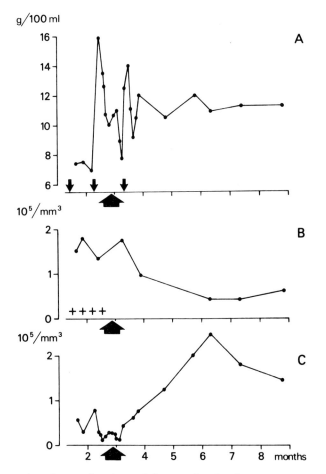

Fig. 1. Evolution of hematological parameters in case No. 1.
A: hemoglobin (g/100 ml). Arrows indicate blood transfusions.
B: reticulocytes (per mm³) (o———o) and immature nucleated cells,
   (+++) in blood.
C: platelets (per mm³).
In A, B and C, larger arrows indicate the bone marrow transplantation.

    In case No. 1 bone resorption was obtained with correc-
tion of hematological abnormalities. The child, a girl, was
born of Saudi Arabian parents after a fullterm pregnancy
without known intake of osteo-condensing agents by the
mother. No other case was recorded in the family. At birth,
weight and size were 2.7 kg and 47 cm. At about 2 months,
abnormal searching eye motions with optic atrophy were already present. Plasma calcium (8.5 mg/100 ml) and daily
calcium urinary output (5 mg) were low. Calcium kinetic
data were typical for osteopetrosis with very low bone ac-
cretion and resorption and increased calcium balance and
intestinal absorption rates. A metabolic acidosis consistent with a renal tubular defect was detected. The 2-year-
old sister was identical for HLA-A, B and D determinants
and for all erythrocytic antigens and immunoglobulin allo-
types tested. She was therefore chosen as a donor. Except

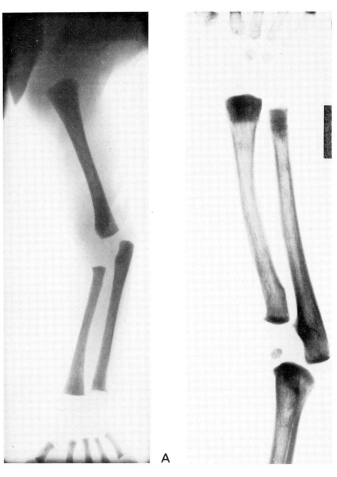

Fig. 2. Case No. 1: X-rays; (a) 2.5 months; (b) 10.5 months.

for vitamin D (400 units/day), no therapy was given to the
child prior to, during or after transplantation. In the
weeks following transplantation, alterations were observed
and are still present 30 months later. At +3 months, the
hepatosplenomegaly had disappeared and the blood picture
was entirely corrected (Fig. 1). X-rays revealed progressive modifications of bone (Fig. 2), mainly the appearance
of medullary cavities with distinct cortex and marrow
space. Dense transverse metaphyseal bands became visible.
The base of the cranium remained dense. Symptoms of optic
atrophy persisted despite an attempt at neurosurgical de-
compression at 7 months of age. Plasma calcium level increased (9.0 mg/100 ml on average). Calcium kinetics indicated a raised bone-accretion rate and a higher calcium
balance than normal. The slowly exchangeable calcium compartment had decreased. Plasma alkaline phosphatase activity decreased (680 mU/ml). Growth and development have pro-

gressed, but size and weight are still below normal (-2 S.D.).
The renal condition remained unchanged. Due to the identity
between the donor and the recipient, no evidence of the
survival of transplanted cells was available.

These observations indicate that a restoration of
bone resorption can be achieved in human osteopetrosis by
transplanting compatible lymphoid cells. This new approach
of the disease was suggested by experimental studies in
animals: major issues are still to be obtained, namely the
demonstration of the nature of effector (=resorbing) cells;
the role of a graft in the persistent bone resorption after
transplantation; the mechanisms involved in resorption (21,
22,23).

In man, despite the fact that all forms of osteopetrosis may not respond and that optimal conditions, especially
the use of preparative immunosuppression, are not yet
defined, cell transplantation may be considered in severe
forms of the disease.

REFERENCES

1. Marks, S.C. and Walker, D.G. (1976): Mammalian osteopetrosis, a
    model of studying cellular and humoral factors in bone resorption.
    In: The Biochemistry and Physiology of Bone, IInd Ed., Vol. IV,
    pp. 227-301. Editor: G.H. Bourne. Academic Press, New York.
2. Walker, D.G. (1973): Osteopetrosis cured by temporary parabiosis.
    Science, 180, 875.
3. Walker, D.G. (1975): Bone resorption restored in osteopetrotic
    mice by transplant of normal bone marrow and spleen. Science, 190,
    784.
4. Walker, D.G. (1975): Control of bone resorption by hematopoietic
    tissues. The induction and reversal of congenital osteopetrosis
    in mice through use of bone marrow and splenic transplants. J.
    exp. Med., 142, 651.
5. Walker, D.G. (1975): Spleen cells transmit osteopetrosis in mice.
    Science, 190, 785.
6. Moutier, R., Toyama, K., Cotton, W.R. and Gaines, J.F. (1976):
    Three successive genes for congenital osteopetrosis in the Norway
    rat. J. Hered., 67, 189.
7. Marks, S.C. (1978): Studies of the cellular cure for osteopetrosis
    by transplanted cells: specificity of the cell type in 'ia' rats.
    Amer. J. Anat., 151, 131.
8. Marks, S.C. (1973): Pathogenesis of osteopetrosis in the 'ia' rat:
    reduced bone resorption due to reduced osteoclast function. Amer.
    J. Anat., 138, 165.
9. Marks, S.C. (1977): Osteopetrosis in the toothless ('tl') rat:
    presence of osteoclasts but failure to respond to parathyroid ex-
    tracts or to be cured by infusion of spleen or bone marrow cells
    from normal littermates. Amer. J. Anat., 149, 289.
10. Moutier, R., Lamendin, H. and Berenholc, S. (1973): Ostéopétrose
    par mutation spontanée chez le rat. Exp. Animals, 6, 87.
11. Toyama, K., Moutier, R. and Lamendin, H. (1974): Résorption os-
    seuse après parabiose chez le rat 'op'. C.R. Acad. Sci. (Paris),
    D, 278, 115.

12. Milhaud, G., Labat, M.L., Graf, B., Juster, M., Balmain, N., Moutier, R. and Toyama, K. (1975): Demonstration cinétique, radiographique et histologique de la guérison de l'ostéopétrose congénitale du rat. C.R. Acad. Sci. (Paris), D, 280, 2485.
13. Moutier, R. and Lamendin, H. (1977): Guérison de l'ostéopétrose par injection de moelle allogénique chez le rat 'op'. C.R. Acad. Sci. (Paris), D, 284, 1697.
14. Milhaud, G., Labat, M.L., Viegas-Pequignot, E., Dutrillaux, B., Moutier, R. and Toyama, K. (1975): Migrations cellulaires au cours de la guérison provoquée de l'ostéopétrose du rat 'op' et thymus. C.R. Acad. Sci. (Paris), D, 281, 1929.
15. Maroteaux, P. (1975): Les Maladies Osseuses de l'Enfant, p. 133. Flammarion, Paris.
16. Fraser, D., Kooh, S.W., Chan, A.M. and Cherian, A.G. (1968): Congenital osteopetrosis, a failure of normal resorptive mechanisms of bone. Calif. Tiss. Res., 2, 52.
17. Ballet, J.J., Griscelli, C., Coutris, C., Milhaud, G. and Maroteaux, P. (1977): Bone marrow transplantation in osteopetrosis. Lancet, 2, 1137.
18. Ballet, J.J. and Griscelli, C. (1978): Lymphoid cell transplantation in human osteopetrosis. Proceedings, Mechanisms of Localized Bone Loss. Editors: J.E. Horton, T.M. Tarpley and W.F. Davis. Calcified Tiss. Abstr., Spec. Suppl., pp. 399-414.
19. Ballet, J.J. and Griscelli, C. (1977): Essai de Transplantation Médullaire dans l'Ostéopétrose Sévère du Nourrisson. Journées Parisiennes de Pédiatrie, Flammarion.
20. Ballet, J.J. and Griscelli, C. (1978): Bone marrow transplantation in osteopetrosis (letter to the Editor). Lancet, 1, 933.
21. Nisbet, N.W., Menage, J. and Loutit, J.F. (1978): Host-donor cellular interactions in the treatment of experimental osteopetrosis. Nature (Lond.), 271, 464.
22. Walker, D.G. (1978): Abbrogation of congenital osteopetrosis by leukocyte subpopulations. Proceedings, Mechanisms of Localized Bone Loss. Editors: J.E. Horton, T.M. Tarpley and W.F. Davis. Calcified Tiss. Abstr., Spec. Suppl., pp. 383-387.
23. Marks, S.C. (1978): Studies of the mechanism of spleen cell cure for osteopetrosis in 'ia' rats: appearance of osteoclasts with ruffled borders. Amer. J. Anat., 151, 119.

IV. Supportive care, isolation, decontamination

THE INFLUENCE OF HLA MATCHING AND LEUKOCYTE CROSS-MATCH TESTS UPON PLATELET TRANSFUSION RESPONSES IN HIGHLY ALLOIMMUNIZED PATIENTS

J. Gmür and A. von Felten

Division of Hematology, Department of Internal Medicine, University Hospital of Zurich, Switzerland

SUMMARY

Twenty-five thrombocytopenic patients refractory to random-donor platelet support were given 106 platelet transfusions obtained from 58 different HLA-typed single-donors. For critical evaluation of the transfusion responses 'fullhouse' HLA-typing of donors and a precise measurement of the number of infused platelets was performed. Post-transfusion platelet increments were related to the HLA-matching of donor-recipient pairs and to in vitro leukocyte cross-match tests. The transfusion response displayed a striking difference depending on the absence (type 0-match) or presence (type 1- or 2-match) of donor HLA antigens differing from the recipient: Whereas 95% of transfusions from type 0-match donors resulted in a compatible platelet increment, only 20% successful transfusion responses could be achieved with type 1- or 2-match donors. In 77% of type 1- or 2-match transfusions with poor post-transfusion platelet increments, the lymphocyte cytotoxicity test (incubation time 180 min at room temperature) was positive. This test therefore seems to be a useful tool in predicting the outcome of transfusion responses in type 1- and 2-match pairs. In contrast, the lymphocyte cytotoxicity tests were of no predictive value in type 0-match pairs. The influence of selective anti-granulocytic antibodies on type 0-match platelet transfusions was assessed in 4 recipients. Although severe transfusion reactions were observed, no detrimental influence on platelet increments could be observed, at least initially.

The incidence of hemorrhage in thrombocytopenic patients with bone marrow aplasia can be reduced by platelet transfusions (1-3). However, multiple transfusions of platelets from unselected, random donors have usually resulted in alloimmunization with subsequent refractoriness to random donor platelet support (4,5). Yankee et al. have shown that such patients will further respond to platelets compatible for the loci A and B of the HLA system (6-8). On the other hand, it has recently been claimed that only 70% of allo-immunized patients do respond to standard platelet concentrates from HLA-identical donors (9,10). But responses in the remaining 30% mostly could be improved by removing contaminating leukocytes in such platelet concentrates (9). Non-HLA antigen-antibody reactions involving platelets as 'innocent bystanders' have been postulated to explain poor post-transfusion platelet increments despite HLA identity (9).

The present study was carried out in patients highly refractory to random donor platelets in order to evaluate (1) the transfusion response of such patients to platelets from single-donors of different degrees of HLA identity, (2) the value of different in vitro leukocyte cross-match tests in predicting the response to single-donor transfusions, and (3) the influence of anti-granulocyte antibodies upon in vivo transfusion response.

MATERIALS AND METHODS

Platelet collection from single-donors was performed by three different methods: (1) by use of the AMINCO CELLTRIFUGE (American Instrument Company, Silver Spring, Md. (11)): 56 collections with a mean of 4.8×10^{11} platelets; (2) by use of HAEMONETIC'S Mod. 30 (Haemonetic Corporation, Natick, Mass. (12)): 36 collections with a mean of 4.1×10^{11} platelets; (3) by the standard 'split-ACD' method (13) preparing two to four consecutive platelet concentrates per donation: 14 collections with a mean of 2.0×10^{11} platelets per donation. For preparation of leukocyte-poor platelet concentrates, an additional centrifugation of 178 x g/3 min was performed before platelet transfusion (9). Platelets were kept at room temperature and administered within 6 hours after collection. In vivo effectiveness of platelets collected by the three different methods proved to be identical as to the 24-hour post-transfusion recoveries in compatible transfusion responses (see also ref. 14).

Platelet counts were done by phase contrast microscopy (15) of the collected platelet concentrates as well as of the recipient prior to and 24 hours after transfusion.

Histocompatibility testing was done by the standard micro lymphocyte cytotoxicity method (16) with antisera detecting 13 HLA-specificities of locus A and 17 of locus B. In all recipients and donors included in this study four HLA antigens of the two loci A and B were defined without exception; homozygosity of either locus was regularly verified by HLA typing of the parents.

Leukocyte cross-match tests between donor white blood cells and pre-transfusion recipient sera were performed simultaneously by two micro lymphocyte cytotoxicity tests ((1) standard incubation time of 60 min at room temperature (standard-LT, 16); (2) incubation time of 180 min at room temperature (long-LT)), as well as by the micro granulocyte cytotoxicity test (GT, 17). All cross-match tests were repeated later on with donor leukocytes being tested simultaneously against the pre-transfusion as well as weekly collected post-transfusion recipient sera.

Absorption studies of the granulocytotoxic antibodies were performed with either granulocytes (10^8/ml serum), lymphocytes ($2.5-5 \times 10^9$/ml), or thrombocytes (5×10^9/ml), each incubated for 10 min at 37^OC followed by 60 min on ice.

150

The recipients of single-donor platelet transfusions
were 6 patients with aplastic anemia and 18 with acute
leukemia, all with pre-transfusion platelet counts below 6
x 10^9/l due to bone marrow failure. All had multiple random
transfusions in their past history leading to refractoriness to further platelet support from random donors as
judged by failure to increase circulating platelet counts
after transfusion of 6 to 10 random platelet concentrates
on at least three occasions. Patients with either fever
over 38°C, sepsis, suspected disseminated intravascular
coagulation or splenomegaly at the time of single-donor
transfusion were excluded from this study.
  Platelet donors were 58 normal healthy adults selected
among family members of the patients or from a computerized
file of over 3,000 ABO- and HLA-typed unrelated blood donors
from the Swiss Red Cross blood banks.
  The transfusion responses were expressed as 'corrected
platelet increments' in order to evaluate the post-transfusion increments independently of size of the recipients
and various doses of transfused platelets. Therefore platelet increments 24 hours after transfusion were multiplied
by body surface area in sq m and divided by the calculated
number of so-called 'platelet units' transfused. One 'platelet unit' being 0.85 x 10^{11} platelets, the number of 'units'
could be calculated from the total number of platelets collected divided by 0.85 x 10^{11}. In accordance with Yankee,
transfusion responses were defined as compatible if the
corrected 24-hour post-transfusion increments were at least
4.5 x 10^9/l x sq m/U (9). All transfusions were ABO and
cross-match compatible.
  Matching of donor-recipient pairs were classified into
3 types according to the number of non-identical HLA-anti-
gens: type 0-, 1- and 2-match, corresponding to zero, one
and two donor antigens differing from the recipient. Twenty-
five patients were supported 106 times with platelets from
58 different donors thus resulting in 58 different donor-
recipient pairs. With respect to our classification to the
HLA matching between donor and recipient, 18 pairs were of
type 0, 21 pairs of type 1, and 19 pairs of type 2. In
addition to responses to the initial transfusion in these
58 different pairs, responses to subsequent transfusions
of the same donor could be analyzed in 11 out of the 18
type 0-match pairs.

RESULTS

Response to the initial transfusion

Results of the initial transfusion of each donor-recipient
pair are depicted on Figure 1. Type 0-match platelet transfusions (left column) were compatible in 17 out of 18 pairs,
with a mean corrected 24 hour increment of 8,300 platelets/
cu mm/U x sq m. Eight pairs were genotypic identical siblings, 4 non-relatives with identical HLA phenotype and in

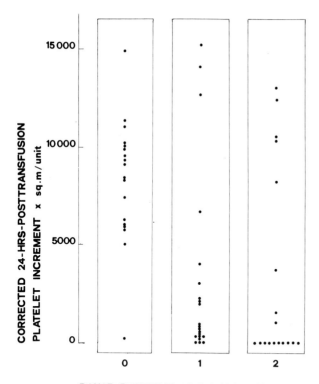

Fig. 1. Corrected 24-hour post-transfusion platelet increments (increment x sq m/'unit') after platelet transfusion of different donor-
recipient HLA match grade in alloimmunized patients (see methods).
Each point represents a single donor-recipient pair.

the remaining 6 pairs non-related donors were homozygous
for HLA locus A and/or B. Transfusion responses of non-
related donors did not differ significantly from those of
HLA identical siblings (mean corrected increment 8,725 versus 7,750). The sole incompatible platelet transfusion originated from a genotypic identical, MLC non-reactive sibling. Type 1-match platelet transfusions (middle column)
were compatible in 4 and incompatible in 17 pairs and type
2-match platelet transfusions (right column) were compatible
in 5 and incompatible in 14 pairs.

Response to repeated transfusions from the same donor in
type 0-match pairs

Repeated transfusions of single-donor platelets were performed in 11 pairs of type 0-match only. In 5 pairs, all
subsequent transfusions (minimum 2, maximum 19, mean 9)
continued to reveal compatible responses. Four of them were
HLA identical, MLC non-reactive sibling pairs, one a non-
related pair. In contrast, in the remaining 6 pairs compatible responses to the initial transfusion shifted to incompatibility after 1 to 3 subsequent transfusions; 1 of
them was a MLC non-reactive sibling pair, 5 were non-

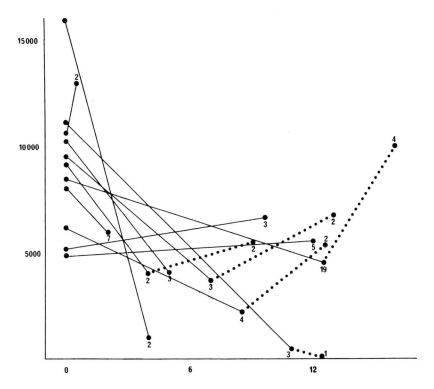

Fig. 2. Corrected 24-hour post-transfusion platelet increments (increment x sq m/'unit') in type 0-match pairs after the initial (left
points) and the final (right points) platelet transfusion of the same
donor. The figures near the final increment in each donor-recipient
pair indicate the number of platelet transfusions given from the same
donor (——— : ordinary single-donor platelet preparations; ······· :
leukocyte-poor single-donor platelet preparations). Abscissa indicates
the time period between initial and final transfusion.

related pairs. However, compatible responses were again
achieved by reduction of contaminating leukocytes in the
platelet preparation in 3 out of 4 type 0-match pairs tested (Fig. 2)..

Correlation of initial transfusion responses and in vitro
leukocyte cross-match tests

The value of in vitro leukocyte cross-match tests in predicting the outcome of platelet transfusion responses was
analyzed in 51 donor-recipient pairs.

a. Lymphocyte cytotoxicity tests

Cross-match tests were performed in 34 type 1- and 2-match
pairs prior to the initial transfusion (Table 1). Eight
pairs with compatible transfusion responses consistently
had negative tests. In 26 situations with poor post-transfusion platelet increments, 20 long-LT were positive,
whereas only 17 showed simultaneously a positive standard-

153

TABLE 1. Transfusion response to the initial single-donor platelet transfusion in type 1- and type 2-match donor-recipient pairs and corresponding in vitro leukocyte cross-match tests (* number of pairs with positive test/number of pairs tested)

Leukocyte cross-match test	Transfusion response	
	compatible	incompatible
Standard-LT+	0 / 8*	17 / 26*
Long-LT+	0 / 8	20 / 26
GT++	2 / 8	14 / 24

\+ Lymphocyte cytotoxicity tests (see methods).

++ Granulocyte cytotoxicity test.

LT. Six tests were false-negative before transfusion, 3 of them converted to positive 7 to 19 days after transfusion.

Pre-transfusion cross-match tests were performed in 17 type 0-match pairs (Table 2). Of the 16 pairs with compatible transfusion responses, 13 had negative tests whereas 3 displayed a positive long-LT, twice in combination with a positive GT. The only incompatible transfusion response was observed in a sibling pair in which a strongly positive long-LT as well as GT was obtained in spite of HLA identity and MLC non-reactivity.

TABLE 2. Transfusion response to the initial single-donor platelet transfusion in type 0-match donor-recipient pairs and corresponding leukocyte cross-match tests (* number of pairs with positive test/number of pairs tested)

Leukocyte cross-match test	Transfusion response	
	compatible	incompatible
Standard-LT+	0 / 16*	0 / 1*
Long-LT+	3 / 16	1 / 1
GT++	6 / 14	1 / 1

\+ Lymphocyte cytotoxicity cross-match test (see methods).

++ Granulocyte cytotoxicity test.

b. Granulocyte cytotoxicity tests

Sixteen type 1- and 2-match pairs showed a positive GT. In 11 of them, standard-LT was also positive; all showed an incompatible transfusion response. The remaining 5 pairs demonstrated an exclusively positive GT; 2 of them had a compatible transfusion response in spite of this positive GT and a high number of contaminating leukocytes in the platelet concentrates (0.8 and 1.1 x 10^9 per transfusion), 3 showed an incompatible response.

Of special interest are 4 type 0-match pairs with an exclusively positive GT. All 4 showed a compatible transfusion response although severe febrile transfusion reactions occurred.

Specificity of granulocyte cytotoxic antibodies

Absorption studies were performed in patients with an exclusively positive GT and compatible transfusion responses. In 3 sera tested, anti-granulocytic antibodies could not be absorbed, neither with a mixture of platelets originating from 120 random donors, nor with platelets and lymphocytes obtained from the respective donors. However, elimination of the antibodies was achieved by corresponding donor granulocytes.

DISCUSSION

To date, no general consensus has emerged concerning the percentage of successful transfusion responses which can be achieved in polysensitized patients, or to what degree HLA specificities should be matched (9,18,20). In order to answer these questions special attention was given to the exact calculation of the number of transfused platelets and to the precise determination of HLA differences between platelet donors and recipients.

According to Yankee et al., transfusion responses may be expressed as post-transfusion platelet increments corrected per sq m of recipient body surface area and per platelet unit infused. The platelet units collected from random donors represent an average of 0.85 x 10^{11} platelets per concentrate (9). However, preparation of multiple units from one single-donor reveals a highly variable number of platelets depending on platelet-count in a donor at the time of collection (14,21). If calculation of corrected increments to single-donor platelets is based only on the average number of platelets usually found in random platelet concentrates (6-9,18), the transfusion responses may be over- or underestimated. Therefore, to calculate platelet increments after transfusion of platelets collected from one donor, the exact number of platelets infused was always determined and expressed in 'standardized units' of 0.85 x 10^{11} platelets.

Furthermore, all platelet donors and recipients whose

155

HLA typing did not reveal two specificities for each of the loci A and B were excluded from this study. Thus, we were able to characterize precisely the grade of HLA match (denoted as type 0-, 1- and 2-match; see methods) in all donor-recipient pairs. Under these conditions, almost 95% of the patients refractory to random-donor platelet support continued to demonstrate good transfusion responses to platelets obtained from type 0-match donors, either MLC non-reactive siblings or unrelated individuals. In contrast to our results it has recently been claimed that only 50 to 70% of polysensitized patients will respond to initial platelet transfusions from 'HLA compatible' single-donors. However, since in that study 'fullhouse'-typing was available in only 71% of matched donor-recipient pairs (9), some of their poor transfusion responses may have been caused by sensitization of recipients to undetected HLA specificities of the donors.

In sharp contrast to the highly successful transfusion responses to type 0-match platelets, our results with donors of type 1- or 2-match were very poor: only 20% of these transfusions produced a platelet increment which could be called compatible, and no significant difference could be observed between donor-recipient pairs with either one or two donor HLA antigens lacking in the recipient. Obviously, the transfusion success using platelets with donor antigens not present in the recipient will depend on the degree of polysensitization of the recipients. Therefore, our patients were selected on the basis of incompatible post-transfusion platelet increments to at least two random-donor transfusions within a few days before performance of the first single-donor transfusion. A much higher rate of compatible transfusion responses to type 1-match donors has been observed by others in bone marrow transplant recipients (18). This could be explained by the extensive immuno-suppressive treatment in connection with bone marrow transplantation (22).

The high proportion of compatible transfusion responses in type 0-match pairs (95%) and the poor responses in type 1- and 2-match pairs (20%) confirm the outstanding role of HLA antigens of locus A and B with respect to platelet support in sensitized patients (6-9). But since the most effective, i.e. type 0-match donors often are not available due to the complexity of the HLA system, sensitive cross-match tests are required to pick out compatible donors of type 1- or 2-match. Compared with various cross-match·tests used (23), lymphocyte cytotoxicity tests meet this demand to a considerable extent, particularly if the incubation time with complement is extended to 180 minutes at room temperature: in 77% of type 1- and 2-match pairs, a poor post-transfusion increment was predicted by a positive test. On the other hand, no false-positive lymphocyte cytotoxicity tests were observed in all 8 compatible type 1- or 2-match transfusions tests. However, in type 0-match pairs with compatible responses, 3 out of 16 tests were false-positive. They could be observed in 2 patients with aplastic anemia who had received excessive numbers of platelet transfusions, prepared firstly from random donors, later on repeatedly from several type 0-match donors. Both developed anti-lymphocytic antibodies which reacted with type 0-match donor lymphocytes, indicating that antigens of other than HLA-A or -B specificity may be involved, e.g. B-lymphocyte allo-antigens not shared by thrombocytes (24). Moreover, antibodies against specificities not being coded for in the major histocompatibility region may occur as well, since in one patient, anti-lymphocyte antibodies were found reacting with cells of his HLA- and MLC-identical sister. Thus, in contrast to type 1- or 2-match pairs, the predictive value of positive lymphocyte cytotoxicity tests applied to type 0-match pairs is questionable.

The role of selective anti-granulocytic antibodies which are accused in the literature of influencing platelet transfusion to a remarkable extent (9) can only be assessed in type 0-match pairs where concomitant influences of HLA antibodies can be excluded. Among our patients, pure anti-granulocytic antibodies were present in four such situations. In all of them, compatible transfusion responses with platelets not deprived of granulocytes were observed at least initially. Thus, antigranulocytic antibodies seem not to influence initial platelet support.

From these in vitro studies, we can conclude that antibodies directed against non-HLA-A or -B antigens do not necessarily cause poor platelet transfusion responses at least initially. However, after repeated platelet transfusions from the same type 0-match donors, transfusion responses may shift to incompatibility. But reduction of contaminating leukocytes in the platelet concentrates can restore compatible responses thus confirming the role of contaminating leukocytes in such situations (9).

REFERENCES

1. Alvarado, J., Djerassi, I. and Farber, S. (1965): Transfusion of fresh concentrated platelets to children with acute leukemia. J. Pediat., 67, 13-22.
2. Freireich, E.J. (1966): Effectiveness of platelet transfusion in leukemia and aplastic anemia. Transfusion, 6, 50-54.
3. Cavins, J.A., Farber, S. and Roy, A.J. (1968): Transfusion of fresh platelet concentrates to adult patients with thrombocytopenia. Transfusion, 8, 24-27.
4. Ster, R.H., Levin, R.H., Cooper, H. and Freireich, E.J. (1964): Complement fixing isoantibodies in serum of transfused persons: Correlation of antibodies with platelet survival in thrombocytopenic patients. Transfusion, 4, 428-435.
5. Shulman, N.R. (1966): Immunological considerations attending platelet transfusion. Transfusion, 6, 39-49.
6. Yankee, R.A., Grumet, F.C. and Rogentine, G.N. (1969): The selection of compatible platelet donors for refractory patients by lymphocyte HLA-typing. N. Engl. J. Med., 281, 1208-1212.

7. Yankee, R.A., Graff, K.S., Dowling, R. and Henderson, E.S. (1973): Selection of unrelated compatible donors by lymphocyte HLA matching. N. Engl. J. Med., 288, 760-764.

8. Lohrmann, H.P., Bull, M.I., Decter, J.A., Yankee, R.A. and Graw Jr, R.G. (1974): Platelet transfusions from HLA compatible unrelated donors to alloimmunized patients. Ann. intern. Med., 80, 9-14.

9. Herzig, R.H., Herzig, G.P., Bull, M.I., Decter, J.A., Lohrmann, H.P., Sout, R.F., Yankee, R.A. and Graw, R.G. (1975): Correction of poor platelet transfusion responses with leukocyte-poor HLA-matched platelet concentrates. Blood, 46, 743-750.

10. Bucher, U., De Weck, A., Spengler, H., Tschopp, L. and Kummer, H. (1973): Platelet transfusions: Shortened survival of HLA-identical platelets and failure of in vitro detection of anti-platelet antibodies after multiple transfusions. Vox Sang. (Basel), 25, 187-192.

11. Graw Jr, R.G., Herzig, G.P., Eisel, R.J. and Perry, S. (1971): Leukocyte and platelet collection from normal donors with the continuous flow blood cell separator. Transfusion, 11, 94-101.

12. Reiss, R.F. and Katz, A.J. (1976): Statewide support of thrombocytopenic patients with ABO matched single donor platelets. Transfusion, 16, 312-321.

13. Technical Methods and Procedures (ed 6), 1974, pp. 186-187. American Association of Blood Banks, Washington, D.C.

14. Gmür, J., Hirvonen, H., Fehr, J. and Honegger, H.P. (1977): Leistungsfähigkeit des Blutzellseparators 'Haemonetic 30' bei der Gewinnung von Plättchen aus Einzelspendern. Schweiz. med. Wschr., 107, 1452-1453.

15. Brecher, G. and Cronkite, E.P. (1950): Morphology and enumeration of human blood platelets. J. appl. Physiol., 3, 365-377.

16. Mittal, K.K., Mickey, M.R., Singal, D.P. and Terasaki, P.I. (1968): Serotyping for homotransplantation. XVIII. Refinement of microdroplet lymphocyte cytotoxicity test. Transplantation, 6, 913-927.

17. Hasegawa, T., Graw Jr, R.G. and Terasaki, P.I. (1973): A microgranulocyte cytotoxicity test. Transplantation, 15, 492.

18. Cornu, P., Groff, P., Weber, W., Nissen, C., Burri, H.P. and Speck, B. (1976): Thrombozytenersatz mit HLA-typisierten nichtverwandten Einzelspendern. Schweiz. med. Wschr., 106, 889-893.

19. Thorsby, E., Helgesen, A. and Gjemdal, T. (1972): Repeated platelet transfusion from HLA compatible unrelated and sibling donors. Tissue Antigens, 2, 397-404.

20. Mittal, K.K., Ruder, E.A. and Green, D. (1976): Matching of histocompatibility (HL-A) antigens for platelet transfusion. Blood, 47, 31-41.

21. Schiffer, C.A., Buchholz, D.H. and Wiernik, P.H. (1974): Intensive multiunit plateletpheresis of normal donors. Transfusion, 14, 388-394.

22. Gluckmann, E., Devergie, A., Marty, M., Faille, A. and Barrett, A.J. (1977): Treatment of severe aplastic anemia with anti-lymphocyte globulin. Exp. Hematol., 5/Suppl. 2, 104.

23. Filip, D.J., Duquesnoy, R.J. and Aster, R.H. (1976): Predictive value of cross-matching for transfusion of platelet concentrates to alloimmunized recipients. Amer. J. Hematol., 1, 471-479.

24. Mann, D.L., Abelson, L., Harris, S. and Amos, D.B. (1975): Detection of antigens specific for B-lymphoid cultured cell lines with human alloantisera. J. exp. Med., 142, 84-90.

158

HLA AND NON-HLA ANTIBODIES INFLUENCING PLATELET TRANSFUSION RESULTS

A. Brand, A. van Leeuwen, J. Langerak, A. Niterink, J.G. Eernisse and J.J. van Rood

Department of Immunohaematology and Blood Bank, University Hospital, Leiden, The Netherlands

Unless special precautions are taken to prepare extremely leukocyte-depleted blood components, almost all patients will develop refractoriness to random platelets after multiple transfusions (1). When the patient becomes sensitized, the usual approach is to look for HLA-matched donors in the family or in a panel of typed volunteers. In case no full-house identical donors are available a lymphocytotoxicity crossmatch is performed with partially matched donors (2,3, 4). The number of failures, however, with this approach is rather high.

We analysed retrospectively 251 combinations, which were divided into 3 degrees of compatibility: A, B and C matches (see legend Table 1). These transfusions were administered to 76 thrombocytopenic patients who were totally refractory to random platelets. Indications for platelet transfusions were either a platelet count lower than 10,000 mm^3 or bleeding. Patients with severe infections or signs of consumption coagulopathy were excluded. A transfusion was judged successful if the 20 hours' increment was over 4500 platelets mm^3 per unit[*] infused, corrected for body surface area.

Table 1 indicated that HLA-matched donors showed a much lower failure rate than mismatched donors, despite the presence of lymphocytotoxic antibodies, which were not detectable against the mismatched antigen or antigens in the C donors. More intriguing is that about 30% of the HLA-matched combinations also showed a poor recovery. From the data in Table 2 it appears that an extensive use of homozygous (B match) donors is fully justified because they gave the same results as 4 antigen-identical unrelated donors. On the other hand, although they did slightly but not significantly better, HLA identical family donors also had a high percentage of failures. It is unlikely that incompatibility for HLA-C is the cause of these transfusion failures because it is in strong linkage disequilibrium with HLA-B. Moreover, the results with HLA identical family donors indicate that the factor or factors causing these transfusion failures are in all probability to be located outside the HLA complex.

---

[*]1 unit is the number of platelets from 500 ml of ACD blood. The in vitro recovery with the extra ACD method is 60-80%.

TABLE 1. Evaluation of transfusion failures of platelet donors selected by HLA type and negative lymphocytotoxicity crossmatch

| | 20 hours' increment/U x BSA | | |
	≥4500	0-4000	% failures
Number of A matches	55	23	29.5
Number of B matches	68	33	32.6
Number of C matches	24	48	66.7
Total 251	147	104	41

A match: all antigens between donor and recipient shared.
B match: no incompatible antigens, the donor is homozygous for the A and/or B antigen(s).
C match: ≥one mismatch, not selected for crossreactive antigens.

TABLE 2. Evaluation of transfusion failures of platelet transfusions of HLA identical or HLA compatible donors

| | 20 hours' increment/U x BSA | | |
	≥4500	0-4000	% failures
Related Number of A matches	34	13	27.7
Unrelated Number of A matches	21	10	32.3
Unrelated Number of B matches	68	33	32.6
Total	123	56	31

Screening of sera of multitransfused patients yielded a very low incidence of positive reactions when tested against platelets (5), although 20 different techniques were used (6,7,8).

Recently good fluorescein-labelled anti-human globulin sera became commercially available and we extended our platelet donor selection procedure with an indirect immuno-fluorescence test on donor platelets. A rabbit (Fab) anti-human IgG (Fc) rhodamine-labelled antibody was used[x] (9). Donor platelets, incubated with autologous serum, served as a control or background value and usually gave a percentage of fluorescent 'cells' of 0-10; this level was subtracted from the crossmatch value. The predictive value of this test was investigated in 27 refractory patients, for whom 118

[x]Nordic, GaHu IgG (Fc) (TRITC) 27-2-74.

combinations of different match grades were selected. In all combinations the lymphocytotoxicity crossmatch between patient's serum and donor lymphocytes was negative.

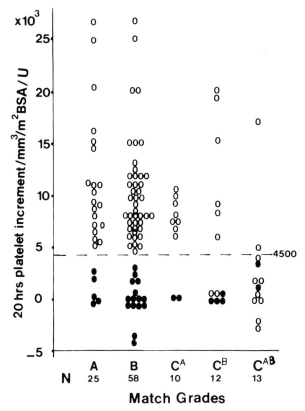

Fig. 1. Twenty hours' increment of 118 selected donor-recipient combinations with a negative lymphocytotoxicity test. o = negative indirect platelet immunofluorescence test. ● = positive indirect platelet immunofluorescence test. A match: all 4 antigens shared. B match: donor homozygous for the A and/or B antigens. C^A: one mismatch for an HLA-A antigen. C^B: one mismatch for an HLA-B antigen. C^{AB}: one haplotype mismatch.

In Figure 1 the corrected 20 hours' increment is shown. Of these combinations, 38 (32%) gave an insufficient increment of less than 4500 platelets/mm³/U. The closed circles mean a platelet crossmatch with ⩾15% fluorescent platelets (net) after incubation with patient's serum. If this test had been taken into account, the number of failures would have been reduced to 10 out of 90 (11%). All these failures of the new donor selection procedure occurred only in combinations with one mismatch for an HLA-B antigen or a haplotype mismatch (see Table 3). We have preliminary indications that the reason for these failures is the variable expression of almost all B antigens on platelets, a phenomenon already known for HLA-B8 and -B12 (10,11). Weak antibodies not able to induce a positive lymphocytotoxicity crossmatch will also be negative in the indirect platelet immuno-fluorescence technique if the donor has a low expression of the corresponding HLA-B antigen on his platelets. Despite the low antigenic density it appears that platelets can be destroyed when antibodies are present. Improvement of the results with HLA-mismatched donors can probably be obtained by using a more sensitive lymphocyte crossmatch, e.g. an indirect lymphocyte fluorescence technique.

TABLE 3. Evaluation of transfusion failures of platelet donors selected by HLA type, negative lymphocytotoxicity crossmatch and negative indirect platelet immunofluorescence test

| | 20 hours' increment/U x BSA | | |
	⩾4500	0-4000	% failures
Number of A matches	20	0	0
Number of B matches	43	0	0
Number of C matches	17	10	37
Total	80	10	11

By combining a lymphocytotoxicity and an indirect platelet immunofluorescence crossmatch we obtained an improved platelet donor selection. Nevertheless, the nature of the antibodies reacting with HLA identical platelets and affecting platelet survival is still unclear.

Although in one patient a platelet specific antibody of the anti-Zw^a type appeared to be present (12), the antibodies in most of the other patients appeared to be directed against lymphocytes. These antibodies were incapable of inducing lymphocytotoxicity. Three observations point in the direction of a non-HLA system, shared between platelets, lymphocytes and probably other cells: (1) Absorption of some of these patients' sera with HLA identical lymphocytes removed the anti-platelet activity. (2) From a group of 68 patients who were regularly transfused with extremely leukocyte-depleted blood and platelets, 75% did not become refractory to HLA antibodies, nor did these non-HLA antibodies occur (13). (3) Preliminary simultaneous testing of these patients' sera against platelets and lymphocytes of the same HLA identical donor in a fluorescence technique showed these antibodies reacting with the donor's B and T lymphocytes.

CONCLUSION

Although anti-HLA antibodies are the main cause of platelet refractoriness, a second system also plays an important role.

162

This appears to be a non-HLA system, present on platelets but also on lymphocytes and probably on other cells. One of the speculations is that the importance of this system has wider implications than just platelet donor selection, if we keep in mind that one of the three bad prognosis factors in the Seattle transplant patients is refractoriness for platelets (14) and that this correlation is still un-explained.

REFERENCES

1. Rejada, F., Bias, W.B., Santos, G.W. and Zieve, P.D. (1973): Blood, 42/3, 405.
2. Bosch, L.J., Eernisse, J.G., van Leeuwen, A. et al. (1965): Rev. belg. Path., 31, 139.
3. Yankee, R.A., Grumet, F.C. and Rogentine, G.N. (1969): New Engl. J. Med., 281, 1208.
4. Yankee, R.A., Graff, K.S., Dowling, J.S. et al. (1973): New Engl. J. Med., 288, 760.
5. Marcelli-Barge, A., Poirier, J.G. and Dausset, J. (1973): Vox Sang. (Basel), 24, 1.
6. Shulman, N.R., Aster, R.H., Leitner, A. and Hiller, M.C. (1961): J. clin. Invest., 40, 1597.
7. Duquesnoy, R.J., Lorentzen, D.F. and Aster, R.H. (1975): Blood, 45/6, 741.
8. Wu, K.K., Hoak, J.C., John, M.D. et al. (1975): New Engl. J. Med., 292, 130.
9. Brand, A., van Leeuwen, A., Eernisse, J.G. and van Rood, J.J. (1978): 51/5, 781.
10. De Mouzon, A., Ohayon, E., Pris, J. and Julien, F. (1976): Vox Sang. (Basel), 31, 58.
11. Aster, R.H., Scatkowski, N., Liebert, M. and Duquesnoy, R.J. (1977): Transplant. Proc., IX/4, 1695.
12. Van der Weerdt, C.M., Veenhoven-Riesz, L.F., Nijenhuis, L.E. and van Loghem, J.J. (1963): Vox Sang. (Basel), 8, 513.
13. Eernisse, J.G. and Brand, A. (1979): J. exp. Hemat., submitted for publication.
14. Thomas, E.D., Fefer, A., Buckner, C.D. and Storb, R. (1977): Blood, 49/5, 671.

INFECTIOUS COMPLICATIONS IN PATIENTS UNDERGOING BONE MARROW
TRANSPLANTATION

T.R. Rogers

on behalf of

The Westminster Hospitals Bone Marrow Transplant Team,
London, United Kingdom

The infectious complications arising in 10 patients undergoing bone marrow transplantations are described. Each patient was managed in strict isolation in a Vickers-Trexler
isolator and decontamination of the skin, mucous membranes
and bowel was performed according to the regime described
elsewhere (1).

RESULTS

The results are summarised in Table 1. It can be seen that
half the patients already had serious infections prior to
isolator entry. Three of these patients died. During the
487 days of isolation 2 (♀ 14 and ♀ 26) developed super-
added fatal infections. However, no infections attributable
to exogenous microorganisms occurred. All infected cases
had received vigorous systemic antimicrobial therapy with
white cell support, when available, from chronic granulocytic leukaemia donors. No prophylactic systemic antibiotics
were given. The patient who developed severe cytomegalovirus
infection is discussed elsewhere in this symposium. The
finding of polyoma virus particles in the urine of 2 of the
patients has been reported (2). One patient (♂ 49), who
had been successfully grafted, later died from gram negative
septicaemia after exit from the isolator. More recently, a
12-year-old male has undergone two marrow grafts; during 22
weeks of tent isolation he developed one episode of strepto-
coccal septicaemia which responded to systemic antibiotic
therapy.

CONCLUSION

While the incidence of infectious complications in this
group is high it is evident that most of these patients had
established infection prior to, or shortly after, coming
under our care. The high fatility in this group emphasizes
the bad prognosis associated with serious infection prior
to grafting.

TABLE 1. Clinical infections before and during treatment in isolator

Patients (yr)	Diagnosis	Days in isolator	Infections pre-entry	Superadded infections
♂ (9)	Aplastic anaemia	4	E. coli septicaemia Anal abscess	–
♀ (14)	Aplastic anaemia	35	E. coli septicaemia	–
♀ (14)	Aplastic anaemia	75	Streptococcal pharyngitis Oral candidiasis	E. coli septicaemia
♀ (16)	Aplastic anaemia	95	–	Cytomegalovirus infection
♀ (26)	Aplastic anaemia	72	–	Systemic candidiasis
♂ (49)	Aplastic anaemia	36	Vibrio parahaemolyticus bacteraemia E. coli septicaemia	–
♀ (5/12)	S.C.I.D.	14	Pseudomonas septicaemia Salmonella enteritis	–
♀ (6/12)	S.C.I.D.	53	–	Lobar pneumonia
♂ (7)	Chronic granulo-matous disease	31	Staphylococcus aureus and Aspergillus osteomyelitis	–
♂ (15)	Fanconi's anaemia	72	–	–

REFERENCES

1. Watson, J.G., Rogers, T.R., Selwyn, S. and Smith R.G. (1977):
   Evaluation of Vickers-Trexler isolator in children undergoing
   bone marrow transplantation. Arch. Dis. Childh., 52, 563-568.
2. Henry, K. (1978): Some ultrastructural aspects of bone marrow
   transplantation: hitherto unrecognized manifestations of GVHR involving heart, and polyoma virus infection in two children. Pathol.
   Biol., 26/1, 55-56.

INFECTIONS IN GRANULOCYTOPENIA. THE EFFICACY OF PARTIAL ANTIBIOTIC DECONTAMINATION[x]

H.F.L. Guiot[1] and J.W.M. Van der Meer[2]

[1]Isolation Ward, J.A. Cohen Institute of Radiopathology and Radiation Protection, Leiden, and [2]Department of Infectious Diseases, University Hospital, Leiden, The Netherlands

SUMMARY

Two groups of granulocytopenic episodes were compared for incidence of infection. The patients in group A were isolated in conventional isolation rooms, the patients in group B were more strictly isolated and received partial antibiotic decontamination (PAD).
   From Group A the following conclusions could be drawn:
a. during 100-500 granulocytes/mm^3 (severe granulocytopenia) life-threatening infections are relatively rare.
b. below 100 granulocytes/mm^3 (extreme granulocytopenia) the number of serious infections rises sharply and mortality is high.
c. the necessity of extensive measures to prevent infections is questionable as long as granulocytes are above 100/mm^3.
   In group B, the mean duration of extreme granulocytopenia per episode was higher than in group A, however, in group B 37.5% of the episodes of extreme granulocytopenia were associated with infection, whereas in group A this percentage was 76.2%. Thus PAD seems to be an effective measure to prevent infection in those patients who are likely to become extremely granulocytopenic.

Infection is the main hazard for the neutropenic patient. There is considerable controversy in the literature about the measures applied to prevent and treat infection (nursing in protected environment, prophylactic antibiotics, choice of antibiotics, granulocyte transfusions, decontamination etc.).
   Recently a method for decontamination - partial antibiotic decontamination (PAD) - was reported (1); the aim of this method is to prevent infection by eradication of the patient's endogenous, potentially pathogenic aerobic flora with preservation of the anaerobic flora of the gut. Anaerobic bacteria are able to diminish colonization by potentially pathogenic strains (2).
   In this paper the morbidity and mortality during granulocytopenic episodes in patients not decontaminated and nursed in a conventional isolation room are compared with

[x]This study was supported in part by the J.A. Cohen Institute of Radiopathology and Radiation Protection.

167

morbidity and mortality during granulocytopenic episodes in patients who were partially decontaminated and more strictly isolated.

METHODS

Treatment

Over the past years our policy in granulocytopenic patients has been as follows (3). No systemic antibiotics are given until bacterial infection is seriously suspected or proven. Granulocyte transfusions are only given to patients with agranulocytosis and proven bacterial infection that does not respond to appropriate antibiotic therapy.

Patients

Patients with less than 500 granulocytes per mm^3, admitted to the wards of the Department of Internal Medicine are nursed in conventional isolation rooms and do not receive PAD. Granulocytopenic patients admitted to the Isolation Ward of our hospital received PAD, sterile food and are semi-isolated (1). Semi-isolation is isolation in a laminar flow isolator with one of the curtains opened over a width of about 80 cm or a comparable system. Protected by a well-fitting mask, the patients are allowed to leave the isolator twice daily, but they do not meet other patients.

The data of a prospective study (performed in the first half year of 1976) on the incidence and outcome of infections in granulocytopenic episodes (Van der Meer, Alleman and Boekhout, submitted for publication) are used in the present paper (episodes in patients with PAD are excluded from this group). This group is referred to as group A. All patients from 1975 up to March 1978 who were partially decontaminated had one or more granulocytopenic episodes; these episodes are referred to as group B.

Partial antibiotic decontamination

PAD was carried out as described earlier (1). In short: the naso-oropharynx is sprayed with an aqueous solution of 3% gentamicin 4 times a day; amphotericin B 3%, neomycin 3%, and cephaloridin 3% contained in Orabase[R] are applied 4 times a day to the mouth to a total of 1 g ointment per day to decontaminate the gastrointestinal tract; capsules containing 250 neomycin, 100 mg polymyxin B and 250-500 mg amphotericin B or miconazole and tablets containing 1000 mg nalidixic acid are given by mouth 4 times a day; the skin is washed daily with povidone-iodine soap and water containing 0.5% chlorhexidine; the prepuce or vulval and vaginal region is treated with a cetylbase-cream containing the same combination of antibiotics as the one used for the mouth.

Classification

a. Infectious status - Proven bacterial and fungal infections were classified as either major (severe) infections or minor infections. Septicemia or organ invasion (e.g. pneumonia, perirectal abscess, meningitis, endocarditis, arthritis, and osteomyelitis) were considered major infections: stomatitis, pharyngitis, skin abscess and sinusitis were classified as minor infections.
b. Granulocytopenia - An episode of granulocytopenia was taken as the number of days during which a patient had less than 500 granulocytes/mm^3. According to the severity of granulocytopenia two groups were distinguished: severe granulocytopenia (100-500 granulocytes/mm^3) and extreme granulocytopenia (less than 100 granulocytes/mm^3).

Microbiology

A bacteriological inventory of the patient's endogenous microflora was carried out as described earlier (1).

RESULTS

In Table 1 the two groups are compared for age and diagnosis. In group A the granulocytopenic episodes concern patients who are relatively older than in group B and there are more granulocytopenic episodes in patients with acute non-lymphocytic leukemia in group A (58.3%) than in group B (44.8%). On the other hand aplastic anemia is more frequent in group B.

TABLE 1. Characteristics of granulocytopenic episodes

		Group A (no PAD)	Group B (PAD)
Age (yr)	mean age	46.5	31
	range	21-71	15-55
Diagnoses			
	acute non-lymphocytic leukemia	21	13
	acute lymphocytic leukemia	4	2
	various myelo- and lympho-proliferative disorders	6	1
	aplastic anemia	3	13
	others	2	-
Total number of episodes		36	29

TABLE 2. Days with infection during granulocytopenia in group A

	0–500 granulo-cytes (total)	100–500 granulo-cytes/mm^3 ('severe granu-locytopenia')	<100 granulo-cytes/mm^3 ('extreme granulocyto-penia')
Total number of granulocytopenic days	1214	750	464
Total number of days with infec-tion	316 (26.0%)	70 (9.3%)	246 (53.0%)
Major infection	229 (18.8%)	47 (6.3%)	182 (39.2%)
Minor infection	87 (7.2%)	23 (3.1%)	64 (13.8%)

In Table 2 the total number of days associated with infec-tion are given for group A and also for episodes of severe granulocytcpenia (100–500 granulocytes/mm^3) and during epi-sodes of extreme granulocytopenia (<100 granulocytes/mm^3). The number of days with infection is low during severe granulocytopenia, but this number is rising sharply (>50%)

TABLE 3. Number of infections during granulocytopenic episodes in group A (no PAD)

	Severe granulocytopenia (100–500 granulocytes/mm^3)	Extreme granulocytopenia (<100 granulocytes/mm^3)
Infection	4	16
major	1	12
minor	3	4
No infection	11	5
Total	15	21

during extreme granulocytopenia. In group A significantly more major infections are seen during extreme granulocyto-penia than during severe granulocytopenia (chi square 7.6, p<0.006) (Table 3) and also mortality due to infection is closely associated with extreme granulocytopenia (Table 4).

The total number of days in group B was 1777. In all episodes of group B, granulocytes fell below 100/mm^3 during a total of 817 days (46%). In contrast with group A, where

170

TABLE 4. Survival and death in granulocytic episodes in group A (no PAD)

	Severe granulocytopenia	Extreme granulocytopenia
Mortality due to infection	0	8
Death due to other causes	1	3
Survival	14	10

maximally one period of extreme granulocytopenia per granu-locytopenic episode occurred, more than one extremely granulocytopenic period was observed during 10 out of the 29 episodes in group B. Thus, in total 40 extreme granulo-cytopenic periods were studied in group B.

The infections and mortality due to infection in group B during extreme granulocytopenia are given in Table 5. In this group 15 of the 40 episodes of extreme granulocytopenia (37.5%) are associated with infection, whereas in group A 16 out of 21 extremely granulocytopenic episodes (76.2%) are associated with infection (see Table 3). For major in-fections these percentages are 25.0 in group B and 57.1 in group A.

TABLE 5. Infections during periods of extreme granulocytopenia in group B (PAD)

Infection	15[x]	
major		10
minor		5
No infection	25	

[x]5 patients died due to infection.

DISCUSSION

In the present paper two groups of patients with granulocy-topenia, treated in the same hospital are compared. The pa-tients in group A were only isolated in conventional isola-tion rooms, the other group was isolated more strictly and was subjected to partial antibiotic decontamination.

The two groups are not comparable for age and diagno-ses. Those patients selected for bone marrow transplantation and/or treatment with anti-thymocyte globulin (4) were ad-mitted to the Isolation Ward and received PAD, which explains the high number of patients with aplastic anemia in group B.

Both groups also differ in duration of extreme granulocytopenia (<100 granulocytes/mm^3): in group A the mean number of days with extreme granulocytopenia per episode was 12.8 and in group B the mean was 20.4. This longer mean period of extreme granulocytopenia in group B probably indicates more serious disease and more aggressive myelosuppressive treatment.

It was found in group A that the number of infections rise very sharply and that mortality increases, when granulocytes fall below 100/mm^3. This leads to the conclusion that extreme granulocytopenia is a very high risk to acquire infection.

In view of the small number of life-threatening infections during severe granulocytopenia, extensive measures to prevent infections seem to be questionable as long as granulocytes are above 100/mm^3. However, for patients who are likely to become extremely granulocytopenic (e.g. patients selected for bone marrow transplantation) measures that may effectively prevent infection are valuable.

Is PAD such a measure? Despite the longer mean period of extreme granulocytopenia, the relative number of infections in group B is lower than in group A. So PAD seems to be effective, and it has advantages over other measures (such as total decontamination, prophylactic granulocyte transfusions, parenteral prophylactic antibiotics): PAD is well tolerated, adverse effects are rare, strict isolation is not needed and it is relatively cheap.

REFERENCES

1. Guiot, H.F.L. and Van Furth, R. (1977): Partial antibiotic decontamination. Brit. med. J., 1, 800-802.
2. Van der Waay, D., Berghuis-de Vries, J.M. and Lekkerkerk-Van der Wees, J.E.C. (1971): Colonization resistance of the digestive tract in conventional and antibiotic treated mice. J. Hyg., 69, 405-411.
3. Nauta, E.H. and Van Furth, R. (1975): Infection in immunodepressed patients, the approach to diagnosis and treatment. Infection, 3, 202-208.
4. Speck, B., Gluckman, E., Haak, H.L. and Van Rood, J.J. (1977): Treatment of aplastic anaemia by antilymphocyte globulin with and without allogeneic bone marrow infusions. Lancet, 2, 1145-1148.

PROGRESS WITH TENT ISOLATORS

James Graham Watson

Westminster Medical School and Children's Hospital, London,
United Kingdom

A description of the way in which we care for transplant
patients in a modified Vickers-Trexler isolator.

The flexible film isolators are situated in general
paediatric wards and the patients are cared for by medical
and nursing staff who have responsibility for other general
paediatric patients. The isolator canopy is hung from light
metal poles and the canopy kept at an automatic positive
pressure using 1415 L/min blower. The ingoing air is passed
through 0.3 μ HEPA filters. The bed is outside the canopy
but all bedding, medical and nursing equipment is inside.
Access to the patient is via built-in flexible plastic
half-suits with clear visors to give an undistorted view.
Each half-suit has an additional air supply to aid the
person working therein. Different sizes of isolator allow
appropriate care for the infant, the toddler and the older
child and also allow aseptic transport of the patient to
other hospital departments.

The isolator is sterilised with peracetic acid initially and thereafter anything entering the isolator must
be sterilised, either by gamma radiation to 2.5 Megarads,
steam autoclaving or hypochlorite disinfection. There is an
entry port through which items can enter the isolator asep-
tically against a positive pressure air flow, and an exit
port, closed by a bag, through which rubbish may be removed,
the technique allowing isolation never to be broken.

Frozen food is sterilised by gamma radiation or else
good quality tinned food is very carefully surface disin-
fected. There is a choice of 23 main dishes and 16 desserts.
A cooker, kettle, toaster and a refrigerator sleeve inside
the isolator allow a wide variety of foods. Most children
receive total parenteral feeding for some time but this is
outside the isolator and directed through a plastic cone
into a central venous line.

Procedures such as lumbar puncture, electrocardio-
graphy, electroencephalography, ultrasound studies and even
a barium meal have all been carried out inside the isolator.

No electronic communication aids are required and
other children in the ward can play games with the tent
occupant. Glove sleeves, if reversed, are used by the child
to adjust television or radio sets. A telephone sleeve is
provided. Parents are actively encouraged to help with

caring for their child.

There is no doubt that the nurses and medical staff feel less isolated from the patient with this form of isolation compared with cubicle isolation and to have the isolator in a ward with other children is helpful to both the isolated patient, his parents and the attending staff.

Over 782 days of exclusion isolator experience with 12 patients, including 487 days with neutrophils less than 500/cu mm and 270 days with neutrophils less than 100/cu mm, there has been only one episode of bacterial contamination which was due to a tear in the visor of a half-suit. Although patients have contracted bacterial infection whilst in the isolator these have, with this one exception, been due to organisms which were known to have entered the isolator tent with the patient despite extensive decontamination.

We have recently used an infant isolator to contain a patient with severe salmonellosis who was a danger to other patients. To convert the isolator from exclusion mode to containment took about 3 hours and the nurses found no difficulty in readapting their techniques.

THE PROVISION OF STERILE DRUGS FOR PATIENTS IN ISOLATORS

Andrew Brown and John Sloggem

Pharmacy Department and Bone Marrow Transplant Team,
Westminster Hospital, London, United Kingdom

It is the policy of the Westminster Hospital's Bone Marrow
Transplant Team that all items which enter patient isolators should be sterile. Where drugs cannot be provided in
a sterile form, e.g. tablets, they are provided in a sterile glass bottle, or disposable plastic presterilised
bottles (normally used for collecting clinical specimens).
Our aim is to provide one day's requirement of drugs at a
time. However, if a need has not been anticipating by the
stock piling of drugs in sterile bottles, unopened manu-
facturer's containers are supplied. Transfer of tablets
into sterile containers is carried out under a laminar
flow hood in the pharmacy. This method of working is similar to that adopted by pharmacists at Hammersmith Hospital
(4). These prepared pharmaceuticals then enter the isolator
by way of a 'dunk bath' where they are totally immersed in
a detergent-hypochlorite solution. This is the method
which we adopt if we have no information on the sterilisation of a drug. If this method is used, it should be remem-
bered that unsterilised mixtures, syrups and other aqueous
solutions are good vehicles for microbiological contamination and should be avoided.

Since the initial patients transplanted at this hospital were all children there was a need to provide sterile
liquids for oral use. The obvious source for this type of
preparation is injectable products since they are readily
available, present few stability problems and also this is
a practice adopted in many children's hospitals. A list of
parenteral preparations which may be given orally appears
in Table 1. However, the use of injections may present some
problems, e.g. the pH of the solution may be very alkaline
and thus the oesophagus may be damaged when they are swal-
lowed. If one is forced to use alkaline solutions they
should be washed down with sterile liquids. The drug concentration may be so low that the administration of a large
volume of fluid is necessary. Additionally, the injection
may be unpalatable, making it difficult to persuade a child
to take the drug. We have attempted to mask any unpleasant
taste by producing a range of flavoured syrups based on
sorbitol. This has the advantage of no pH change on autoclaving. However, these have not been used since, in practice, sterile orange juice has been found to be a suitable

175

TABLE 1. Injections which can be administered orally

Calcium gluconate
Chlorpheniramine
Cimetidine
Cyclophosphamide
Diazepam
Digoxin
Disopyramide
Frusemide
Hydrocortisone (as phosphate)
Metoclopramide
Oxprenolol
Phenobarbitone
Phenytoin (freeze dried product only)
Pyrimethamine
Trimeprazine
Vitamin B, Co and C
Vitamin K_1

vehicle.

Adults and older children receiving adult doses do not pose the same problems as paediatric patients, i.e. dosage must be flexible and in a liquid form. It is therefore feasible to consider the use of tablets and capsules for these patients and so the problems involved in their sterilisation must be investigated.

Theoretically the best method of sterilisation is autoclaving, since under standard conditions (i.e. 121°C for 15 minutes) this will reduce a given microbiological population by a greater degree than other available methods. However, this cannot be used when there is no water present and therefore is of little use for dry powders, tablets or suspensions. The latter should be avoided since the core of the suspended particles may be dry and hence not sterilised by this process. This means that this method should be used only for liquids which are stable at autoclaving temperatures (115°C for 30 minutes or 121°C for 15 minutes).

The other commonly used method of sterilisation is membrane filtration, with aseptic precautions, which usually entails passing the liquid through a 0.2 μ (0.2 nm) membrane filter. This method does not have anything like the safety factor of autoclaving and should only be used if other methods are inapplicable. It is also difficult to apply to viscous solutions, e.g. paracetamol syrup. This problem may be overcome by using a small (100 ml) pressure vessel. Filtration cannot be applied to drugs which are unstable in solution, unless the solutions are used immediately.

However, filtration still does not solve the problems posed by tablets, dry powders or suspensions. These, in theory, could be sterilised by dry heat. However, there are few compounds which can withstand the high temperatures (160°C for 60 minutes) necessary for this method of sterilisation. To avoid these problems we investigated gamma radiation as a method of sterilisation. This has the advantage that it penetrates all parts of a dosage form (e.g. tablets or suspensions) and allows sterilisation in the final container. This is a more certain method of sterilisation than aseptic handling. Also in the doses used (2.5 Megarad) there is no increase in the temperature of the substance being irradiated, therefore, thermolabile substances may be sterilised by this method. This method has proved very useful and Table 2 lists those drugs which have been successfully irradiated. The information contained in this Table has been obtained either from published literature (1-3) or from pharmaceutical companies who have been kind enough to analyse gamma irradiated products.

TABLE 2. Drugs which can be sterilised by gamma irradiation

Allopurinol	Miconazole cream
Aluminium hydroxide	Nalidixic acid
Amphoteracin B (lozenges, suspension and tablets)	Neomycin
	Neo-naclex K tablets (bendrofluazide and potassium chloride)
Ampicillin	Niferex (polysaccharide iron complex)
Asilone (Antacid)	Nitrofurantoin
Bonjela	Norethisterone tablets
Cephalexin	Nystatin cream (Dome)
Cephaloridine	Polymyxin B sulphate
Cephradine	Prednisolone tablets soluble
Colistin	Propranolol tablets
Cotrimoxazole tablets (Septrin, Bactrim)	Quinoderm cream (benzoyl peroxide 10%)
Diazepam tablets	Rifampicin
Erythromycin	Senokot tablets
Flucloxacillin	Soframycin
Flucytosine	Sulphafurazole
Fusidic acid	Sulphapyridine
Glycerin suppositories	Ticarcillin
Hydrocortisone acetate	Vancomycin
Kaolin poultice	Vitamin C
Metronidazole	

This information applies to non-sterile dry forms only except where stated.

Gamma sterilisation can produce free radicals which in turn cause oxidation, reduction or hydrolysis of the drug. These are the reactions which drugs normally undergo, hence the standard quality control tests should be valid. If, however, unexpected breakdown products occur they may not be identified by these methods.
Little is known of the effect which sterilisation by gamma irradiation has on the long-term stability of a preparation. In practice, creams and gels cannot be sterilised

by this method. Any exceptions, e.g. Nystatin Dome, must be positively proved to be able to withstand this treatment. Commercially, ointments, e.g. eye ointments, have been sterilised by this method. Because of this lack of information on long-term stability it is good practice for only one month's stock to be kept. This allows ample time for replacement of stock if the patient is in the isolator for a longer period.

Often where gamma sterilisation cannot be applied (see Table 3) there is either a sterile injection or an aqueous formulation which can be sterilised, e.g. multivitamin injection, chlorhexidine solutions.

TABLE 3. Drugs which cannot be gamma irradiated

Chlordiazepoxide
Chlorhexidine
Clonazepam
Creams (some exceptions)
Flavours
Many vitamin preparations
Nitrazepam

When autoclaving, dry heat, sterilisation by filtration or by gamma irradiation cannot be applied the method described by the British Pharmacopoeia (5) of heating with bactericide may be used. This requires heating at 99°C for 30 minutes and we have applied this method to chlorhexidine dental gel (see Table 4), the chlorhexidine in the formulation acting as the bactericide. Table 4 also contains details of a number of miscellaneous products which we have provided for use in the isolators. None of these have been sterilised by gamma irradiation.

TABLE 4. Other preparations available

Chlorhexidine dental gel
Chlorhexidine mouthwash
70% ethanol (for tent cleaning)
Hydrogen peroxide mouthwash 20 vol.
Linoleic acid (use intralipid)
Lithium chloride
Mineral supplement
Sterile water (tap water for drinking or distilled for other uses)

We feel that because of the reduced immunological response of most patients in isolators the provision of sterilised drugs is an essential part of their overall treatment. Wherever possible sterilisation should be by autoclaving, dry heat, or heating with a bactericide. Aseptic filtration or gamma sterilisation should be used only when no other method is practical.

The pharmaceutical companies who have helped us with this work wish to make it clear that they cannot accept any legal responsibility for the information given, though of course it is given in good faith.

REFERENCES

1. Association of British Pharmaceutical Industry (1960): Use of gamma radiation sources for the sterilisation of pharmaceuticals. A.B.P.I., London.
2. Blackburn (1975): Personal communication.
3. Fleurette,J. et al. (1974): Activité bactériostatique de différents antibiotiques après irradiation par rayons gamma. International Atomic Energy Symposium, Bombay. IAEA-SM-192/15, Vienna.
4. Day, A. (1975): Pharmaceutical aspects of a leukaemia unit. Pharm. J., 214, 255.
5. British Pharmacopoeia (1973): Her Majesty's Stationary Office, London.

STUDIES OF CYTOMEGALOVIRUS IN DONORS AND RECIPIENTS

R.S. Pereira, T. Rogers and J.G. Watson

Westminster Hospital Marrow Transplant Team, London,
United Kingdom

SUMMARY

Screening of HLA-matched donor panels for CMV antibody status has revealed groups with higher than expected numbers of antibody carriers;
this is tentatively linked in this population with HLA-BW15. A case of
systemic CMV infection due to transfusion following marrow transplantation is described, with details of successful treatment with adenine
arabinoside.

In the course of screening several 'panels' of volunteer,
HLA-matched but otherwise unrelated donors in connection
with a marrow transplant programme, it was noted that 2
panels, both sharing the tissue type HLA-BW15, had higher
than average numbers of individuals (9/10 and 3/4) with
antibodies to CMV. On further testing of donors possessing
this tissue type, CMV antibodies were found in 16 out of
22 (73%). The donor population was drawn from healthy adults
in the Greater London area, and the frequency of CMV antibody for all the donors so far tested was 49%, which is
comparable to the 54% reported for an age-matched population
examined in London in an earlier survey (see Table 1) (1).
    The 22 donors (mean age 35.3 years) with the tissue
type HLA-BW15 (16 of whom were CMV antibody-positive) were
compared with the 60 donors (mean age 34.1 years) possessing
other tissue types (24 of whom were CMV antibody-positive),
in a Fisher exact probability test, one-tailed since the
direction of the difference was predicted in advance. The
analysis indicated a low probability (P = 0.009) that the
different frequencies of CMV antibody were due to chance
alone.
    The findings suggest that normal donors with tissue
type HLA-BW15 either have greater susceptibility to CMV infection or respond more readily with antibody production
than does the general population. A similar association in
the mouse between CMV susceptibility and the murine major
histocompatibility complex has recently been reported (2).
    Thus, in some transplant cases it may be difficult to
provide CMV-free donations from unrelated donor panels. Two
of our recent cases with this 'susceptible' tissue type
have been infected post-graft by transfusion of fresh

180

TABLE 1. HLA-BW15 and cytomegalovirus antibody

	CMV antibodies			
	+	−	% positive	P[x]
HLA-BW15 (22)	16	6	73	<0.01
Other HLA (60)	24	36	40	N.S.
All donors (82)	40	42	49	N.S.
Stern and Elek[xx] (199)	108	91	54	N.S.

[x]Fisher exact probability test (one-tailed).

[xx]See References (1).

(irradiated) blood products. One was asymptomatic; the other had a severe clinical syndrome with systemic CMV infection and graft-versus-host disease. The latter case was treated successfully with adenine arabinoside (Vidarasine) and will be described in more detail.

A 15-year-old female with severe idiopathic aplastic anaemia received a bone marrow graft from her histocompatible 11-year-old sister. She was managed in strict protective isolation. Eleven days post-graft, she developed fever, diarrhoea, elevated hepatic enzymes and a haemorrhagic morbilliform rash. Skin biopsy showed evidence of graft-versus-host disease for which she was given antilymphocyte globulin. This was followed by clinical improvement but slow haematological recovery.

Forty-five days after grafting, pyrexia recurred, with mental confusion, jaundice and severe diarrhoea, but no evidence of interstitial pneumonia. There was a significant elevation of serum antibody to CMV. However, despite strong clinical suspicion of CMV infection, no chemotherapy was administered until virus was isolated from culture of her peripheral blood white cells in human embryonic lung tissue (see Fig. 1).

She was given a course of adenine arabinoside in a dose of 15 mg/kg/day which was discontinued on the 8th day due to suppression of the total leucocyte count and reticulocyte count. The chemotherapy resulted in cessation of virus growth after the last day of treatment, and subsequently the white cell count recovered to satisfactory levels. Eight months post-graft she was re-admitted to hospital with fever and mild jaundice. The CMV IgG antibody titre, which had been progressively rising, was now 1:32,000, with virus-specific IgM antibodies present. However, attempts at demonstrating the virus by electron microscopy of the urine and cultures of urine, stools, white cells and from the oropharynx proved unrewarding. She was managed conservatively and her symptoms resolved with eventual recovery.

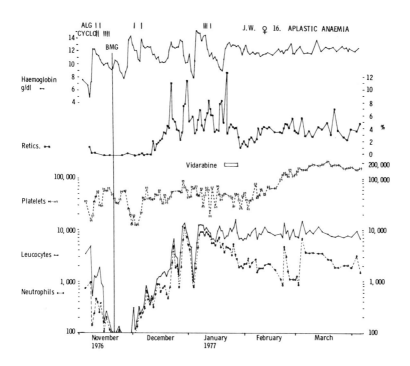

Fig. 1.

Adenine arabinoside is a relatively new antiviral
agent. Although early trials have indicated that it may be
effective in the treatment of human CMV infections (3),
doubt has recently been cast on its efficacy in such cases
(4). Its successful rise in our patient, in producing clinical recovery, suggests that it may be valuable even during
the emergence of a marrow graft. Although there was undoubt-
ed myelosuppression, the graft was not ablated and recovery occurred following cessation of therapy. The recurrence
of symptoms, with a markedly raised antibody titre, suggests
that despite the chemotherapy, virus was not eradicated
even though it was not demonstrated in tissue culture. It
is most likely that she acquired her infection from fresh
blood products, as many of these were positive on retrospective screening for CMV antibody; neither the patient
nor the marrow donor had serological evidence of previous
CMV infection. Her susceptibility to infection may have
been further increased by the antilymphocyte globulin given
post-graft.

In view of this hazard, we would advocate the exclusive
use of CMV-negative donors of blood and blood products in
susceptible cases, although this may be difficult, as suggested above. The similarity in clinical presentation between graft-versus-host disease and systemic CMV infection,
and the possibility of their simultaneous occurrence,

182

emphasise the importance of screening for both conditions concurrently, especially as their respective management is quite different. The use of adenine arabinoside has produced encouraging results in this single case, but it is recommended that haematological monitoring during administration be performed daily and the drug be discontinued at the first sign of marrow suppression; the graft should ideally be well established rather than in an early emergent phase. Nevertheless, the frequency and morbidity of cytomegalovirus infection in marrow graft cases justifies stringent measures for avoidance of infection; where these measures fail, the problems of chemotherapy are not insuperable.

REFERENCES

1. Stern, H. and Elek, S.D. (1965): J. Hyg. (Lond.), 63, 79.
2. Chalmer, J.E., Mackenzie, J.S. and Stanley, N.F. (1977): J. gen. Virol., 37, 107.
3. Ch'ien, L.T. et al. (1974): J. infect. Dis., 130, 32.
4. Editorial (1977): Brit. med. J., 1, 1048.

V. Antilymphocyte globulins

COMPARATIVE STUDIES WITH ANTI-HUMAN-THYMOCYTE GLOBULIN PREPARATIONS PRODUCED IN DIFFERENT ANIMAL SPECIES

J.G. Kreeftenberg, M.F. Leerling, M.E.M. Geleijnse, B.C. Kruijt, J. Nagel and E.J. Ruitenberg

Rijks Instituut voor de Volksgezondheid, Bilthoven, The Netherlands

In order to establish an optimum protocol for the production of anti-human-thymocyte globulin (ATG) we tested the influence of animal species. For this purpose antisera were produced in sheep, goats and horses according to methods published by Monaco (1) and Kelly (2). Rabbits were immunized according to a scheme developed in our institute (3). Sera were compared with regard to their immunosuppressive potency as estimated in a skin graft survival test.

Two animal systems were used to investigate which animal species was suitable for the production of anti-thymocyte serum (ATS). First, the rat was studied as a test model; next, a monkey model with Cynomolgus monkeys. On the basis of the results obtained in the animal models, procedures for the preparation of anti-human ATG were selected.

The results obtained with the anti-rat and anti-Cynomolgus ATS are summarized in Tables 1 and 2. It is obvious that the rabbit produced the most potent antisera in both systems. Furthermore, it was demonstrated that rabbit ATS induced a strong lymphophenia in the monkey. The superior quality of goat ATS as reported by Kelly (2) could not be confirmed.

Based on these results anti-human-thymocyte sera were produced in horses and rabbits. Again the rabbit proved to be the species of choice. These experiments resulted in a routine procedure which has been used for the past 2 years to produce anti-human ATG in rabbits. The consistency of this production method is demonstrated in Table 3. The hematological effects of our rabbit anti-human ATG in the Cynomolgus monkey model is shown in Figure 1. It is concluded that this rabbit anti-human ATG induces a strong and long-lasting lymphopenia with a minor effect on the number of red cells and platelets.

Based on these data different ATG preparations, which are currently used in clinical trials in Europe, were compared. Horse anti-human ATG 1 and 2 were obtained from Dr. M. Bonneau (Lyon) and Dr. B. Speck (Basel). Rabbit anti-human ATG 7 was produced in the Rijks Instituut voor de Volksgezondheid (Bilthoven). In particular the in vivo and in vitro immunosuppressive and toxic activities of the different ATG preparations were studied. A summary of the most important data is given in Table 4.

TABLE 1. Comparison of horse, sheep, rabbit and goat for the production of anti-rat-thymocyte serum

Animal	Serum	Cytotoxicity	Skin graft survival time[x] (days)
Horse	1338	640	7(7- 7)[xx]
	1271	1250	9(8- 9)[xx]
Sheep	147	640	14(9-21)
	148	1250	13(9-20)[xx]
	175	2500	24(11-30)[xx]
	176	2500	21(8-30)[xx]
Rabbit	3794	5000	26(8-30)
	642	2500	28(20-30)
	640	2500	30(29-30)
Goat	38	1250	10(9-10)
	39	1250	8(7- 9)

[x]10 rats were treated with 5 s.c. injections of 1/2 ml serum at days -3, 0, +2, +4 and +7, mean value and range are mentioned. [xx]The rats were treated with 1 ml instead of ½ ml per injection.

TABLE 2. Comparison of horse, sheep, rabbit and goat for the production of anti-Cynomolgus-thymocyte serum

Animal	Serum	Cytotoxicity titer	Number of lymphocytes x 10^6/l		Skin graft survival time[x] (days)
			Day 2	Day 7	
Horse	1274	5000	1800	2590	14 - 15
	1316	2500	670	1400	23 - 23
Sheep	86	10000	2860	1480	16 - 16
Goat	37	10000	1400	1170	14 - 16
Rabbit	492	5000	550	220	42 - 45
	333	1250	130	530	38 - 38
	3388	2500	200	270	42 - 42
	357	2500	480	100	33 - 32

[x]Cynomolgus monkeys were treated with 4 s.c. injections of 8 ml serum/kg at days -3, 0, +2, and +5. The survival time of both skin grafts are mentioned.

All the ATG preparations were stable and contained ≥ 95% immunoglobulin. Furthermore none of the ATG preparations contained significant amounts of endotoxin, antiglomerular basement membrane antibodies, or antibodies against human serum protein. Taking into consideration the protein concentration, the 3 ATG preparations do not differ very

TABLE 3. Immunosuppressive potency of different lots of rabbit anti-human ATG preparations

ATG lot	Cytotoxicity titer[x]	Anti red cell titer[x]	Anti platelet titer[x]	Skin graft[xx] survival time (days)
4	2500	16	< 2	18 - 21
5	2500	4	4	23 - 26
6	2500	4	4	21 - 23
7	1250	8	4	19 - 23
ATS 8[1]	1250	4	4	19 - 23
NRG [2]	< 20	< 8	< 4	8 - 8

[x]Titers were determined in a solution of 5 mg Ig/ml. [xx]Cynomolgus monkeys were treated with 4 s.c. injections of 100 mg Ig/kg at days -2, 0, +2 and +5. The survival times of both skin grafts are mentioned. [1]Unpurified anti-thymocyte serum. [2]Normal rabbit Ig.

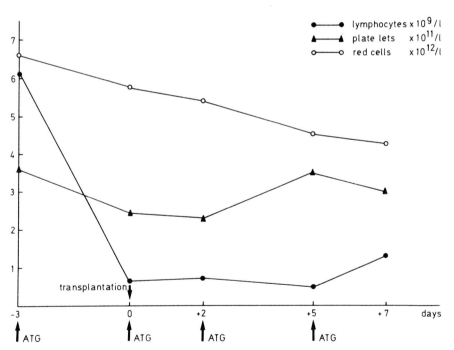

Fig. 1. Hematological data of Cynomolgus monkeys after treatment with an immunosuppressive dose of rabbit anti-human ATG. (Mean values of 10 monkeys with a skin graft survival time ⩾15 days.)

TABLE 4. Summary of the in vivo and in vitro activities of anti-human ATG preparations from different origin

Test models	ATG preparations		
	Rabbit ATG 7	Horse ATG 2	Horse ATG 1
ACTIVITY			
In vitro anti-lymphocyte cytotoxicity	640	2500	1250
immunofluorescence	5000	20000	6400
rosette inhibition	800	1600	1600
In vivo skin graft survival time (days)[x]	19-24	10-12	10-10
Lymphopenia $\dfrac{\text{day } 2+7}{2} \times 10^6/1$	590	2720	3230
SAFETY anti red cell (agglutination)	8	32	128
anti granulocyte (immunofluorescence)	2500	10000	6400
anti platelet (complement fixation)	4	32	32
anti platelet (immunofluorescence)	320	3200	800
PROTEIN conc. mg/ml	5	50	20

[x]The Cynomolgus monkeys were treated with 4 s.c. injections of 100 mg Ig/kg following the scheme indicated in Figure 2.

much in their in vitro activities against lymphocytes, red cells and platelets.

There are, however, striking differences in vivo. In these experiments each ATG preparation was tested in 2 Cynomolgus monkeys which were treated with 4 s.c. injections of 100 mg ATG/kg body weight on days -2, 0, +2 and +5. Two skin grafts from 2 different donors were transplanted on each monkey on day 0. Of each pair of monkeys the results of one monkey are summarized in Figure 2. Both horse ATG 1 and 2 induced a minor decrease in the number of lymphocytes and a slight prolongation of the skin graft survival time of 10-12 days in comparison with 8 days for the control. However, the rabbit ATG 7 induced a skin graft survival time of 19-24 days.

To interpret these findings it has to be mentioned that the Cynomolgus monkey is less sensitive than the Rhesus monkey which is commonly used to measure the immunosuppressive potency of anti-human ATG. With regard to the toxicity, all ATG preparations showed a minor influence on the number of red cells and platelets. Furthermore, the horse ATG 1 and ATG 2 both induced a local reaction such as swelling at the injection site and general reactions, including depression and loss of appetite. Only one monkey treated with ATG 1 showed no adverse reactions. In none of the monkeys could

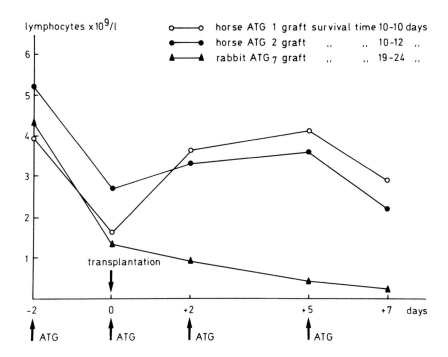

Fig. 2. Immunosuppressive potency of different ATG preparations in Cynomolgus monkeys.

histopathological effects of the ATG treatment on kidney and liver be demonstrated.

In conclusion it can be said that these results confirm our own observations and those reported by Kayhoe (4) that highly immunosuppressive ATG can be produced in rabbits. The availability of such sera may be important as, in a recent paper, F. Thomas (5) reported that only a very strong immunosuppressive rabbit ATG improved the 1.5-year graft survival time of cadaver renal transplants from 42% to 78%.

REFERENCES

1. Monaco, A.P., Wood, M.L. and Russel, P.S. (1967): Some effects of purified heterologous anti human lymphocyte serum in man. Transplantation, 5, 1106.
2. Kelly, G.E., Sheil, A.G.R. and Mears, D.C. (1973): A comparison of in vitro, immunosuppressive and clinical effects of goat and horse anti human thymocyte globulin in Macaca monkeys. Clin. exp. Immunol., 13, 585-594.
3. Kreeftenberg, J.G., Leerling, M.F., Kruijt, B.C. and Geleijnse, M.E.M. (1975): Bereiding en controle van antilymfocyten sera. Ber. Rijks Instituut Volksgezondheid, 33/34, 69-73. (Liber amicorum R. Gispen.)

4. Kayhoe, D.E., Darrow, C.C. and Scott, R.C. (1972): The in vivo activity of antilymphocyte serum. Behring Inst. Mitt., 51, 12-14.
5. Thomas, F., Thomas, J., Flora, R., Mendez-Picon, G., Peace, K. and Lee, H.M. (1977): Effect of antilymphocyte globulin potency on survival of cadaver renal transplants. Prospective randomised double blind trial. Lancet, 2, 671.

THE RELATIVE TOXICITIES OF DIFFERENT PREPARATIONS OF ANTI-LYMPHOCYTE GLOBULIN[*]

M.Y. Gordon and A.J. Barrett

Department of Biophysics, Institute of Cancer Research, and Department of Haematology, Royal Marsden Hospital, Belmont, Sutton, Surrey, United Kingdom

SUMMARY

Different preparations of antilymphocyte globulin (ALG) show widely divergent effects on bone marrow granulopoietic colony-forming cells. Their activities against lymphocytes, assessed by lymphocytotoxicity testing, tended to be more uniform and they were not toxic to mature granulocytes.

   Absorption with acute leukaemic myeloblasts reduced the myelotoxic effect but did not alter the lymphocytotoxic activity.

   Characterisation, in vitro, of different preparations or batches of ALG showed to be useful in selecting the best available for clinical treatment.

Antilymphocyte globulin (ALG) has been used in bone marrow transplantation, both as a conditioning agent for the graft and in the prophylaxis and treatment of graft-versus-host disease (GVHD). Recently, it has been evaluated as a single agent in the treatment of aplastic anaemia.

   ALG may cause marrow suppression and some preparations inhibit bone marrow colony-forming cells (CFU-C) in vitro (1,2,7). A marrow suppressive action of ALG is particularly undesirable when treating patients with aplastic anaemia and patients who have received bone marrow grafts. While it is possible to absorb out this myelotoxicity (8,10) such preparations are not generally available. Some means of selecting non-myelotoxic batches of commercially available ALG would therefore be useful.

   For this reason, we have compared 4 preparations of ALG for their myelotoxicity, using a bone marrow colony assay, and also measured their granulocytotoxicity and lymphocytotoxicity.

MATERIALS AND METHODS

Antilymphocyte globulins (ALGs)

The German (Hoechst), French (Mérieux) and Swiss (Lymphosa)

[*]The work was funded by a grant from the Medical Research Council.

preparations were raised in horses and the Dutch preparation was raised in rabbits. The German and French preparations were obtained from the manufacturers (Hoechst and Mérieux); the Swiss preparation was kindly provided by Dr. Speck and the Dutch ALG was a generous gift from Dr. Kreeftenberg.

Bone marrow colony assay

Buffy coat cells from normal human marrow were washed and plated in agar over leucocyte feeder layers (9). Lysed rat erythrocytes (2.5%) were included in the overlay (7). The plates were incubated at 37°C in a gassed (10% CO_2 in air) humidified atmosphere and colonies of more than 50 cells counted 10 days later.

Myelotoxicity of ALG

Washed bone marrow cells were incubated in gassed, sealed culture tubes in the presence of ALG and 20% autologous serum (as a source of complement) at 37°C for 1.5 hours. The cells were then diluted and plated as above.

Lymphocytotoxicity of ALG

1×10^6 normal lymphocytes, separated from peripheral blood using Lymphoprep, were incubated in Terasaki plates with 0.1 ml rabbit complement and dilutions of ALG for 1.5 hours. Cell viability was assessed using Lissamine green.

Granulocytotoxicity of ALG

Normal granulocytes were separated from peripheral blood using Lymphoprep and the ALGs tested for granulocytotoxicity on papain-treated cells according to the method of Drew et al. (4).

Absorption with leukaemic blasts

Cryopreserved blast cells from patients presenting with acute myeloid leukaemia (AML) were obtained from Dr. R.L. Powles. The method used has been described by Barrett et al. (2). The ALGs were absorbed overnight with 10^8 cells/mg globulin, resuspended and absorbed for a further 1 hour. The cells were then removed by centrifugation.

RESULTS

Figure 1 shows the survival of normal bone marrow colony-forming cells after 1.5 hours' incubation with the ALGs in the presence of complement (autologous serum). Less myelotoxicity was observed when the autologous serum had been heated to inactivate complement (data not given). These ALGs had a wide range of myelotoxic effects from the mild

194

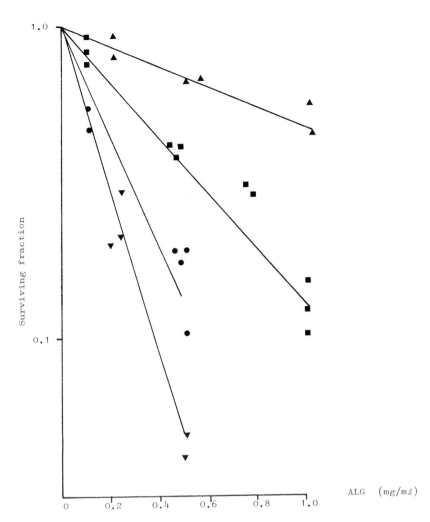

Fig. 1. Effects of ALGs on colony formation by normal human bone marrow cells. ▲ Dutch, ■ French, ● German, ▼ Swiss.

toxicity of the Dutch rabbit preparation to the much greater toxicity of the Swiss preparation.

After absorption with AML blast cells, the toxicities against colony-forming cells were reduced in all cases (Fig. 2). The Dutch and French preparations showed very little toxicity after absorption, but absorption of the German and Swiss preparations did not remove the effect completely.

The results of the granulocytotoxicity assays are given in Figure 3. In no case did the cytotoxicity meet the criterion of Drew et al. (4) who define more than 50% cell kill as a positive result. These measurements were made at 100 μg/well as higher concentrations of the ALGs agglutinated the granulocytes. Measurements on the Swiss preparation were precluded by agglutination even at low concentrations.

Table 1 gives the concentrations of the ALGs required

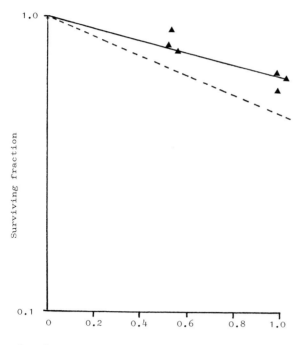

Fig. 2A.   ALG (mg/mℓ)

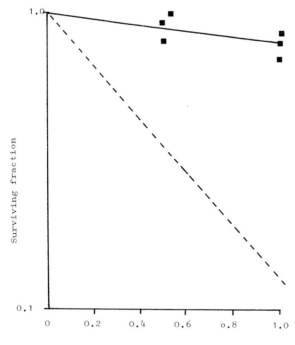

Fig. 2B.   ALG (mg/mℓ)

196

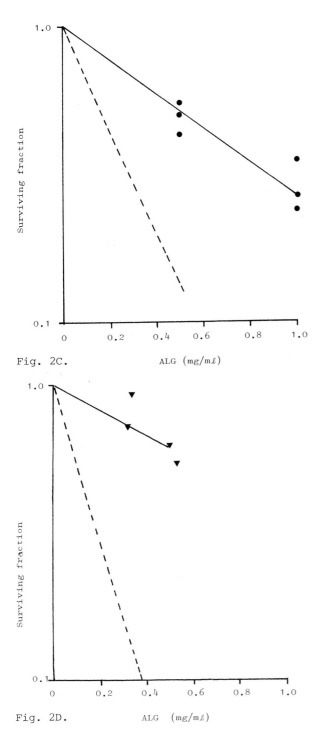

Fig. 2C.

ALG (mg/mℓ)

Fig. 2D.

ALG (mg/mℓ)

Fig. 2. Effects of absorbed ALGs on colony formation by normal human bone marrow cells. ▲ Dutch, ■ French, ● German, ▼ Swiss. ----- effects of unabsorbed preparations.

197

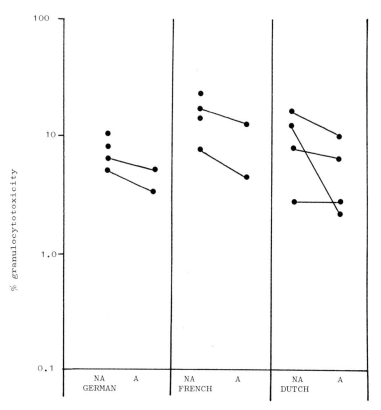

Fig. 3. Granulocytotoxicities of 3 preparations of ALG. NA = pre-absorption. A = post-absorption.

to give 50% lymphocytotoxicity. Three of the ALGs were very similar in their activities against lymphocytes but a greater concentration of the Dutch rabbit preparation was required to give 50% cell kill. Absorption with AML blast cells did not alter the lymphocytotoxic activity.

TABLE 1. Concentration of ALG required to give 50% lymphocytotoxicity

ALG	μg/ml
German	40.0
Dutch	83.4
French	33.3
Swiss	36.6

DISCUSSION

Antilymphocyte globulin (ALG) inhibits human bone marrow colony formation in vitro (2,7,10), and this paper extends earlier observations to a comparison of different preparations of ALG.

Two points have emerged from this study. Firstly the

198

data show that the ALGs tested were not equal in their lymphocytotoxic and myelotoxic effects and indicate that the least myelotoxic (Dutch) ALG was only half as effective as the other preparations when tested for lymphocytotoxicity. It seems reasonable to suggest, therefore, that any selection of ALG should be based on their activities against both lymphoid and myeloid cells and that dosage may need to be adjusted according to the results. Secondly, much higher doses of ALG were required to inhibit colony formation by 50% than were required to achieve the 50% level of lymphocytotoxicity or inhibition of rosette formation. However, even a slight reduction of marrow precursor cells may be clinically significant when the marrow reserve is small and this result cannot be taken to indicate that the myelotoxicity of ALG is unimportant. Indeed, Storb et al. (12) and Barrett et al. (1) have attributed failure of graft take to the administration of ALG to certain patients with aplastic anaemia.

Absorption with myeloid leukaemia cells is effective in removing the myelotoxic effect, confirming the results of Barrett et al. (2). The large numbers of cells required for this simple procedure make it unlikely to be of value in producing therapeutically useful amounts of absorbed ALGs. However, it may be possible to incorporate the cells into immuno-absorbent columns which would be re-used and would reduce the problem of shed leukaemia antigens in the absorbed preparations (13). At the present time it seems better to select the least myelotoxic ALG than to absorb out this effect using myeloid leukaemia cells.

The toxicity of ALG towards the pluripotent haemopoietic stem cell remains the major cause for concern. Although the in vitro colony-forming cell cannot be assumed to reflect the properties of the stem cell in man, there is evidence to suggest that the latter population is also sensitive ALG. The suggested role of ALG in preventing graft take in aplasia (1,12) implies an effect at the stem cell level. Furthermore, studies in animals have shown that the stem cell in animals is inactivated by ALG (3,5). It remains uncertain whether removal of myelotoxicity at the level of the colony-forming cell will produce an ALG without anti-stem cell activity particularly since these 2 populations are thought to be antigenically different (6).

ACKNOWLEDGEMENTS

We wish to thank Miss V.B. Shepherd and Miss T.S. Poole for their excellent technical assistance. V.B.S. and T.S.P. are supported by the Bud Flanagan Fund of the Royal Marsden Hospital.

REFERENCES

1. Barrett, A.J., Humble, J.G. and Hobbs, J.R. (1975): Bone marrow suppression by antilymphocytic globulin. Brit. med. J., 2, 541.

2. Barrett, A.J., Longhurst, P., Rosengurt, N., Hobbs, J.R. and Humble, J.G. (1978): Crossreaction of antilymphocyte globulin with human granulocyte colony-forming cells. J. clin. Path., 31, 129.

3. De Meester, T.R., Anderson, N.D. and Shaffer, C.F. (1968): Effect of heterologous anti-lymphocyte serum on mouse hemopoietic stem cells. J. exp. Med., 127, 731.

4. Drew, S.I., Bergh, O., McClelland, J., Mickey, R. and Terasaki, P.I. (1977): Antigenic specificities detected on papainized human granulocytes by microgranulocytotoxicity. Transplant. Proc., 9, 639.

5. Field, E.O. and Gibbs, J.E. (1968): Cross-reaction of antilymphocyte serum with haemopoietic stem cells. Nature (Lond.), 217, 561.

6. Golub, E.S. (1972): Brain associated stem cells antigen: an antigen shared by brain and haemopoietic stem cells. J. exp. Med., 136, 369.

7. Gordon, M.Y. (1978): Circulating inhibitors of granulopoiesis in patients with aplastic anaemia. Brit. J. Haemat., 39, 491.

8. Mosedale, B., Smith, M.A. and Courtenay, J.S. (1967): Preparation and characterisation of antithymocyte serum and globulin without stem cell activity. Transplantation, 22, 122.

9. Robinson, W.A. and Pike, B.L. (1970): Colony growth of human bone marrow cells in vitro. In: Haemopoietic Cellular Proliferation, p. 249. Editor: F. Stohlman. Grune and Stratton, New York.

10. Rodt, H., Netzel, B., Brehm, G. and Thierfelder, S. (1975): Production of antibodies specific for human thymus-derived lymphocytes purified from antibodies cross-reacting with colony-forming cells. Blut, 29, 416.

11. Rodt, H., Netzel, B., Niethammer, D., Korbling, M., Gotze, D., Kilbe, H.J., Thiel, E., Haas, R.J., Fliedner, T.M. and Thierfelder, S. (1977): Specific absorbed antithymocyte globulin for incubation treatment in human marrow transplantation. Transplant. Proc., 9, 187.

12. Storb, R., Gluckman, E., Thomas, E.D., Buckner, C.D., Clift, R.A., Fefer, A., Glucksberg, H., Graham, T.C., Johnson, F.L., Lerner, K.J., Nieman, P.E. and Ochs, H. (1934): Treatment of established human graft-versus-host disease by antithymocyte globulin. Blood, 44, 57.

13. Zola, H. (1978): Immunoabsorbents prepared from cell membrane antigens: efficiency of incorporation and shedding of protein during use. J. immunol. Methods, 21, 51.

POTENTIAL USEFULNESS OF HETEROLOGOUS ANTILYMPHOCYTE GLOBU-
LINS AND OF ANTI-HLA-DR ALLOANTIBODIES IN HUMAN BONE MARROW
TRANSPLANTATION

J.-L. Touraine, M. Bonneau, E. Gluckman, J. Brochier, J.P.
Revillard and J. Traeger

Unité INSERM 80, Hôpital E. Herriot, Lyon; Institut
Mérieux, Lyon; and Centre Hayem, Hôpital St. Louis, Paris,
France

Graft-versus-host disease remains one of the major hazards
in human bone marrow transplantation. When donor and recipient are matched for the major histocompatibility complex,
the severity of this complication is somewhat reduced. Not
infrequently, however, fatal graft-versus-host disease
still occurs following a bone marrow transplant from an
HLA identical family donor. One of the approaches investigated, in an attempt to reduce the incidence and severity
of graft-versus-host disease, has been the use of hetero-
antisera to eliminate T lymphocytes or of anti-HLA-DR alloantisera which inhibit the mixed leukocyte reaction in
vitro. In this report we describe the preparation and potential use of such antisera.

PURIFIED ANTILYMPHOCYTE GLOBULINS

Horse antilymphocyte serum has been prepared on a large
scale by immunization with thymocytes and thoracic duct
lymphocytes, followed by absorption with polymerized placental tissue. The antilymphocyte globulins (ALG) were
further purified by batch chromatography on QAE Sephadex.
The IgG_2 subclass thus obtained has been previously shown
to retain most of the in vitro antilymphocyte activities
of the total serum. It exerts potent immunosuppressive effects in vivo when injected in low protein concentration to
monkeys or to humans and the resulting immunodeficiency is
predominantly a T-cell deficiency (1).
    The efficacy of ALG in human bone marrow transplanta-
tion is supported by the results of several studies (2-4).
The most convincing evidence of the potency of rabbit anti-
thymocyte globulins in such circumstances is provided by
the beneficial effects observed in patients with already
established and relatively severe graft-versus-host disease
(3). Confirmatory data have been obtained in the treatment
of graft-versus-host disease, with the IgG_2 fraction of
horse ALG by one of us (E.G.). Use of large doses of purified ALG can therefore be recommended to treat established
graft-versus-host disease. Its routine and immediate use at
the time of the transplant, in an attempt to prevent rejec-

tion or graft-versus-host reaction, should however remain
a cautious one as it may somewhat hinder the take of the
graft, even when using batches devoid of demonstrable in
vitro marrow toxicity. In the mouse, prevention of mortality due to acute graft-versus-host disease could be obtained using Fab fragments of ALG which did not appear to
significantly damage hematopoietic stem cells (5).

SPECIFIC ANTI-T LYMPHOCYTE SERA

Rabbit anti-T lymphocyte sera were prepared by immunization
with either human thymocytes or peripheral T lymphocytes
from patients with X-linked agammaglobulinemia. The antisera were rendered specific for T lymphocytes by absorption
with erythrocytes, B lymphoblasts from cultured cell lines,
chronic lymphatic leukemia cells and 'adherent cells'. The
specificity was verified in various assays (6) and the complex systems of antigens recognized by such antisera were
denominated human T lymphocyte differentiation antigens
(HTLA) (7). In 1974 we proposed that such anti-HTLA sera
might be used for in vitro treatment of the bone marrow
graft and would prevent the acute graft-versus-host disease
by removing all cells with a HTLA$^+$ phenotype (6). Since
then, we have observed that most batches of anti-HTLA sera
prepared as described above had little or no toxicity for
CFU-C. However, in order not to interfere with hematopoietic reconstitution, it would seem wise to add a further
absorption stage to remove any possible antibody cross-
reacting with colony-forming cells (8,9). The use of such
anti-HTLA sera, devoid of any anti-CFU-C activity, has already led to very encouraging results in various species,
including man (8-10). As expected, the hematopoietic reconstitution without severe acute graft-versus-host disease,
observed in the first cases thus treated, is comparable to
the reconstitution induced in mice with allologous bone
marrow treated with anti-Thy-1 alloantisera (11-13).

ANTI-HLA-DR ALLOANTIBODIES

The preparation of placental globulins with specificities
against HLA-DR determinants has been previously described
(14-19). Alloantibodies were obtained by elution from a
pool of placental tissues. They were purified and concentrated by ethanol fractionation and batch chromatography.
The IgG preparation, as the F (ab')2 fragments, had in
vitro inhibitory effects on EA rosette formation and on the
mixed leukocyte reaction. The predominantly anti-HLA-DR
activities had been demonstrated on lymphocyte subpopulations, including B-cell-enriched lymphocytes (16). Some
anti-HLA A, B and C activities, however, were found and, to
absorb out those activities, incubation with platelets was
required. Recent use of such preparations in recipients of
kidney transplants has not shown any significant toxicity.
The efficacy cannot, however, be assessed as yet. The use

202

cells. Brit. J. Haemat., 29, 416-426.

9. Mosedale, B., Smith, M.A. and Courtenay, J.S. (1976): Preparation and characterization of antithymocyte serum and globulin without stem cell activity. Transplantation, 22, 122-131.

10. Rodt, H., Netzel, B., Niethammer, D., Körbling, M., Götze, D., Kolb, H.J., Thiel, E., Haas, R.J., Fliedner, T.M. and Thierfelder, S. (1977): Specific absorbed antithymocyte globulin for incubation treatment in human marrow transplantation. Transplant. Proc., 9, 187-191.

11. Cantor, H. (1972): The effects of anti-theta antiserum upon graft-versus-host activity of spleen and lymph node cells. Cell. Immunol., 3, 461-469.

12. Tyan, M.L. (1973): Modification of severe graft-versus-host disease with antisera to the θ antigen or to the whole serum. Transplantation, 15, 601-604.

13. Korngold, R. and Sprent, J. (1978): Lethal graft-versus-host disease after bone marrow transplantation across minor histocompatibility barriers in mice. Prevention by removing mature T cells from marrow. J. exp. Med., 148, 1687-1698.

14. Bonneau, M., Latour, M., Revillard, J.P., Robert, M. and Traeger, J. (1973): Blocking antibodies eluted from human placenta. Transplant. Proc., 5, 589-592.

15. Bonneau, M., Brochier, J., Robert, M., Dubernard, J.M., Fayol, A., Blanc, N., Revillard, J.P. and Traeger, J. (1977): Préparation, propriétés et essais pré-cliniques de gammaglobulines éluées à pH acide à partir de pools de placentas humains. In: Transplantation and Clinical Immunology, pp. 150-163. Editors: J.L. Touraine, J. Traeger and R. Triau. Simep-Editions Publ., Villeurbanne, France.

16. Brochier, J., Bonneau, M., Robert, M., Samarut, C., Revillard, J.P. and Traeger, J.: Anti-HLA-DR alloantibodies eluted from human placental tissue. Transplant. Proc., in press.

17. Revillard, J.P., Brochier, J., Robert, M., Bonneau, M. and Traeger, J. (1976): Immunologic properties of placental eluates. Transplant. Proc., 8, 275-279.

18. Jeannet, M., Faulk, W.P., Creighton, W.D. and Fournier, K. (1973): Blocking of mixed lymphocyte cultures by IgG eluted from human placenta. In: Proceedings, 8th Leukocyte Culture Conference, pp. 243-248. Academic Press, New York.

19. Riggio, R.R., Saal, S.D., Stenzel, K.H. and Rubin, A.L. (1977): Passive immunological enhancement: Biological immunosuppression using retroplacental (maternal) source gamma globulin. In: Transplantation and Clinical Immunology, pp. 140-149. Editors: J.L. Touraine, J. Traeger and R. Triau. Simep-Editions Publ., Villeurbanne, France.

20. Smit, J.A., Myburgh, J.A. and Gaillard, V.J. (1978): Active enhancement in the primate by bone marrow. I. Ia-like determinants on nucleated bone marrow cells. Transplantation, 26, 73-75.

of these globulins is even more preliminary in bone marrow
transplantation and although no marrow toxicity has been
clinically apparent, cautious administration should still
be recommended because of (a) the contaminating anti-HLA,
B and C antibodies in the unabsorbed preparation and (b)
the unknown effect of anti-HLA-DR antibodies on the various
categories of marrow cells expressing HLA-DR antigens (20).
If the lack of marrow toxicity is confirmed and if the pre-
ventive or therapeutic effect of placental globulins on
graft-versus-host disease is established, their systematic
use at the time of transplantation might be worth considering in view of the good clinical tolerance. Furthermore,
the postulated original mode of action should stimulate
studies in the search for a possibly synergistic effect
with various immunosuppressants including ALG.

The use of antisera in bone marrow transplantation is
still at the beginning but results already obtained in
several animal models and in humans are very encouraging.
This field of research is further expected to expand and
to lead to more precise mitigation of both rejection and
graft-versus-host disease, as a result of the preparation
of more narrowly defined antisera or of monoclonal antibodies.

REFERENCES

1. Bonneau, M., Touraine, J.L. and Traeger, J. (1977): Préparation
    et propriétés d'IgG$_2$ antilymphocytaires absorbées. In: Trans-
    plantation and Clinical Immunology, pp. 132-139. Editors: J.L.
    Touraine, J. Traeger and R. Triau. Simep-Editions Publ. Villeur-
    banne, France.
2. Amiel, J.L., Mathe, G., Schwarzenberg, L., Schneider, M., Choay,
    J., Trolard, P., Hayat, M., Schlumberger, J.R. and Jasmin, C.
    (1970): Les greffes de moelle osseuse allogénique après condi-
    tionnement par le seul sérum antilymphocytaire dans les états
    d'aplasie médullaire. Presse méd., 78, 1727-1734.
3. Storb, R., Gluckman, E. and Thomas, E.D. (1974): Treatment of
    established human graft-versus-host disease by antilymphocyte
    globulin. Blood, 44, 57-75.
4. Speck, B., Gluckman, E., Haak, H.L. and Van Rood, J.J. (1977):
    Treatment of aplastic anaemic by antilymphocyte globulin with and
    without allogeneic bone-marrow infusions. Lancet, 2, 1145-1148.
5. Richie, E.R., Gallagher, M.T. and Trentin, J.J. (1973): Inhibition
    of the graft-versus-host reaction. II. Prevention of acute graft-
    versus-host mortality by Fab fragments of antilymphocyte globulin.
    Transplantation, 15, 486-491.
6. Touraine, J.L., Touraine, F., Kiszkiss, D.F., Choi, Y.S. and Good,
    R.A. (1974): Heterologous specific antiserum for identification
    of human T lymphocytes. Clin. exp. Immunol., 16, 503-520.
7. Touraine, J.L. (1975): Human T-lymphocyte differentiation anti-
    gens. Israel J. med. Sci., 11, 1348-1356.
8. Rodt, H., Netzel, B., Brehm, G. and Thierfelder, S. (1975): Pro-
    duction of antibodies specific for human thymus-derived lympho-
    cytes purified from antibodies cross-reacting with colony forming

VI. Graft-versus-host disease

ATTEMPTED CHARACTERIZATION OF THE T-CELL SUBSET RESPONSIBLE
FOR THE INDUCTION OF GVHR

J.-L. Touraine, M.B. Gojon, J. Navarro, C. Genin, R. Fal-
chetti, F. Touraine and O. de Bouteiller

Unité INSERM 80, Hôpital E. Herriot, Lyon, France

A graft-versus-host reaction (GVHR) occurs in 60-70% of
recipients of bone marrow transplants, despite close HLA
matching, and it causes death in 10-20% of them. In laboratory animals, GVHR has been one of the most intriguing and
rewarding models for the analysis of interactions of lymphocyte subsets in vivo. Thus, in clinical transplantation as
well as in basic immunology, GVHR represents a cornerstone
for the understanding and mitigation of allogeneic responses. In the present report we summarize some experimental results which, if interpreted in the context of our
present knowledge, may provide information on the cells
responsible for the induction of GVHR. For the sake of
brevity and clarity we shall limit ourselves to an over-
simplified and schematic representation of the main cell
subsets involved. A more detailed description of interactions between these cells will be published elsewhere.

MATERIALS AND METHODS

As our purpose was to obtain information applicable to GVHR
following lymphocyte administration into immunologically
compromised patients, we chose the model of lethally irradiated mice injected with allogeneic lymphocytes, in pre-
ference to the model of hybrid animals injected with
lymphocytes from an inbred parent.
    Lethally irradiated, 4-week-old female CBA mice were
injected intraperitoneally with lymphoid cell suspensions
from C57Bl/6 mice or from syngeneic mice as controls. The
systemic GVHR was quantified, using the spleen assay (1).
At day 8, mice were sacrificed and the splenic index was
determined. The splenic index is the quotient of the experimental spleen weight divided by the host's body weight
over the control spleen weight (from a syngeneic cell-
injected littermate) divided by its body weight. With this
assay, the minimal splenic index to demonstrate a GVHR was
1.30.
    The injected allogeneic cells were either thymocytes in
certain experiments, or spleen cells in others. They had
been treated in a number of ways: incubation for 4 hours
with thymosin (fraction 5), then washed before injection,
similar incubation but followed by injection without

washings, elimination of PHA-responsive cells by a 3-day culture with PHA and treatment with BUdR and light (2).

In other experiments the injected cells were spleen cells from 'nude' (nu/nu) mice incubated with thymosin (fraction 5) or with a control medium.

RESULTS AND DISCUSSION

Although many cells from different lineages provided both by the donor and the recipient are implicated in the expression of a GVHR (for review, see 3), it has been convincingly demonstrated that inducing cells are T lymphocytes. When lymphoid cells from thymectomized animals were injected into appropriate recipients, no demonstrable GVHR was induced (4). Alternatively, when T lymphocytes were killed by anti-Thy-1 antiserum in the presence of complement, GVHR was also prevented (5).

It soon became apparent, however, that T cells of various origins had very different capabilities to induce a GVHR. More importantly, a cooperation between distinct T-cell subsets was strongly suggested by the synergistic effect of lymph node cells from young and old NZB mice or by the synergism of thoracic duct lymphocytes and cells from other lymphoid organs (6). An interaction between 2 varieties of T lymphocytes, T_1 (present in the thymus and the spleen) and T_2 (present in the peripheral blood and lymph nodes) was then envisioned (7). It was also found that spleen cells induced relatively more splenomegaly than killing, whereas the reverse occurred with peripheral blood or lymph node lymphocytes. A further complexity was introduced by the recognition that certain T lymphocytes may exert a suppressive effect (8) on the mixed leukocyte reaction (MLR), in vitro phenomenon which correlates, at least in part, with the recognition and the proliferative phases of the GVHR.

More recently, the discovery of functionally distinct T-cell subsets recognized by differential expression of Ly differentiation alloantigens has shed some light on the different T-cell subpopulations involved in various responses, including allogeneic responses. From the Ly 123^+ T cells derive 2 cell subsets: The Ly 23^+ T cells which include cytotoxic cell precursors and suppressor cells, and the Ly 1^+ T cells with helper functions (9). In addition, the recognition of determinants coded for by genes of the major histocompatibility complex (MHC) appears to be the following: Ly 23^+ cells are mainly responsive to 'SD' determinants while Ly 1^+ cells proliferate in response to 'LD' determinants.

In a simplified representation of cell interactions, one can therefore envision the pre-cytolytic T cell recognizing certain MHC antigens and being helped in its response by another T cell which recognizes other MHC determinants of the same allogeneic cell. GVHR is indeed amplified when donor lymphocytes and recipient cells differ at both the SD and the LD levels. However, other antigenic systems may stimulate the GVHR-inducing T cells, as shown by the existence of GVHR in MHC-identical pairs. The suppressor T cells exert their inhibition effects on either one of the 2 cooperating T cells (Fig. 1). Comparable information has been obtained in completely in vitro models where evidence for these 3 types of cells has been obtained (10).

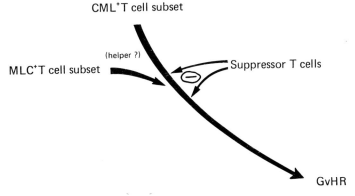

Fig. 1. Schema of the 3 main T-lymphocyte subsets involved in GVHR. The CML$^+$ or cytolytic T cell cooperates with the MLC$^+$ T cell which is responsible for the proliferative phase of GVHR and may exert a helper effect. The suppressor T cell exerts its inhibitory activity on either one of the two other cells.

   In an attempt to further characterize the GVHR-inducing T cells, we made some investigations on their capability to respond to thymic factors. Spleen cells from C57B1/6 mice were incubated with thymosin, then injected into lethally irradiated CBA mice. When the cells were washed after 4 hours of incubation, and before injection, no increase of GVHR was noticed. When the cells were not washed and the thymosin injected with the cells, the GVHR was significantly amplified (Fig. 2). When thymocytes were used in the place of spleen cells and were injected with thymosin, the GVHR was similarly increased (Fig. 3). Experiments using spleen cells from nude mice did not demonstrate induction of GVHR in the allogeneic irradiated recipients. They failed to show any significant GVHR even when cells were incubated and injected with thymosin. Whatever their precise target cell, thymic factors therefore appear to have the capability to amplify the GVHR, provided that there are cells which have already undergone the first stages of T lymphocyte differentiation in the cell suspension injected. The very subset of cells which is mainly responsible for this effect cannot be easily determined in such experiments, especially as the effect was only significant when thymosin was injected in the host with the cells. The influence of thymosin on the recipient's cells which participate in the GVHR can certainly not be excluded or underestimated.

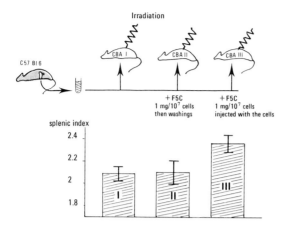

Fig. 2. Influence of thymic factors on the GVHR induced by allogeneic spleen cells injected into irradiated recipients. F5C = thymosin fraction 5 prepared from calf thymuses.

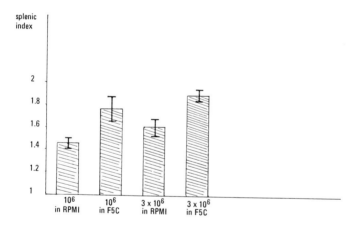

Fig. 3. Influence of thymic factors on the GVHR induced by allogeneic thymocytes injected into irradiated recipients.

In previous in vitro experiments with human lymphocytes, we obtained evidence that T lymphocytes proliferating in response to allogeneic cells were distinct from those responding to phytomitogens (2) and that the latter cell subset had a suppressive effect on the former (11). It was thus felt of interest to determine in the above-described mouse model whether PHA-responsive T cells were different from GVHR-inducing T cells. Spleen cells were stimulated with PHA, treated with BUdR and light, and injected into lethally irradiated allogeneic recipients. The determination of splenic indices in the various groups of mice showed that

210

the inactivation of PHA-responsive cells did not result in a decrease of the GVHR (Fig. 4). This result suggests that the helper T cells, and perhaps also the cytotoxic T cells, involved in the GVHR, do not belong to the subpopulation of T lymphocytes which proliferate in response to PHA. The GVHR was even significantly enhanced after inactivation of PHA-responsive cells (Fig. 4) and one of the possible explanations for this effect postulates the presence of cells with a spontaneous suppressor activity for allogeneic responses among phytomitogen-sensitive cells.

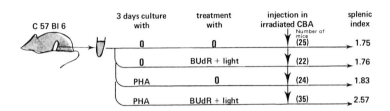

Fig. 4. Separation of PHA-responsive cells from GVHR-inducing cells. Spleen cells from C57Bl/6 mice were cultured for 3 days with PHA or control medium. Some cultures were treated with BUdR and light to inactivate proliferating cells. The cells were then injected intraperitoneally into lethally irradiated CBA mice. The splenic index was determined in the 4 groups of 22-35 mice. It was increased at a significantly higher degree in the 4th group than in the others (p<0.001).

The adaptation of these results to our model of human T lymphocyte differentiation is schematized in Figure 5. This representation, still tentative in its design, awaits further experimental evidence and is merely introduced here to stimulate investigations along these lines to prove or disprove its validity. If confirmed, several means of manipulating the various T-cell subsets might result in a specific mitigation of the GVHR.

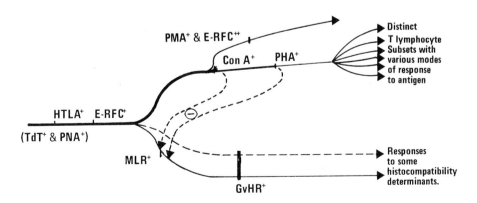

Fig. 5. Schematic representation of some stages of T cell differentiation in man.

REFERENCES

1. Simonsen, M. (1962): Graft versus host reactions. Their natural history, and applicability as tools of research. Progr. Allergy, 6, 349-467.
2. Touraine, J.L., Touraine, F., Hadden, J.W., Hadden, E.M. and Good, R.A. (1976): 5-Bromodeoxyuridine-light inactivation of human lymphocytes stimulated by mitogens and allogeneic cells: Evidence for distinct T-lymphocyte subsets. Int. Arch. Allergy, 52, 105-117.
3. Grebe, S.E. and Streilein, J.W. (1976): Graft-versus-host reactions: A review. Advanc. Immunol., 22, 119-221.
4. Good, R.A., Dalmasso, A.P., Martinez, C., Archer, O.K., Pierce, J.C. and Papermaster, B.W. (1962): The role of the thymus in development of immunologic capacity in rabbits and mice. J. exp. Med., 116, 773-798.
5. Cantor, H. (1972): The effects of anti-theta antiserum upon graft-versus-host activity of spleen and lymph node cells. Cell. Immunol., 3, 461-469.
6. Cantor, H. and Asofsky, R. (1970): Synergy among lymphoid cells mediating the graft-versus-host response. II. Synergy in graft-versus-host reactions produced by Balb/c lymphoid cells of differing anatomic origin. J. exp. Med., 131, 235-246.
7. Cantor, H. and Asofsky, R. (1972): Synergy among lymphoid cells mediating the graft-versus-host response. III. Evidence for interaction between two types of thymus derived cells. J. exp. Med., 135, 764-779.
8. Gershon, R.K. and Leibhaber, S.A. (1972): The response of T cells to histocompatibility-2 antigens. Dose response kinetics. J. exp. Med., 136, 112-127.
9. Cantor, H. and Boyse, E.A. (1975): Functional subclasses of T lymphocytes bearing different Ly antigens. J. exp. Med., 141, 1376-1389 and 1390-1399.
10. Sundharadas, G., Sopori, M.L., Hayes, C.E., Narayanan, P.R., Alter, B.J., Bach, M.L. and Bach, F.H.: Differentiation of precursor cytotoxic T lymphocytes following alloantigenic stimulation. Cold Spring Harbor Symposia on Cell Proliferation, in press.
11. Touraine, J.L. (1978): A model of sequential differentiation and ontogeny of T lymphocytes in man. In: Human Lymphocyte Differentiation: Its Application to Cancer, INSERM Symposium 8, pp. 93-100. Editors: B. Serrou and C. Rosenfeld. Elsevier/North-Holland Biomedical Press, Amsterdam.

SKIN ANTIBODIES PRODUCED BY HUMANS AFTER A BONE MARROW GRAFT REACT WITH EPIDERMAL CELL DIFFERENTIATION ANTIGENS[*]

J.H. Saurat[1], E. Gluckman[2] and L. Didierjean[1]

[1]Clinique Dermatologique et Laboratoire de Pathologie Expérimentale, CHU Necker-Enfants Malades, and [2]Clinique des Malades du Sang, Hôpital Saint-Louis, Paris, France

SUMMARY

Antibodies reacting with the cytoplasm of keratinocytes (KCA) have been found to be produced frequently after a bone marrow graft. Using substrates in which keratinocytes were involved in distinct types of differentiation we have demonstrated that KCA react with cytoplasmic components linked with the stage and the type of keratinocyte differentiation. Stratified squamous epithelia thus appear to be made of several sets of keratinocytes, the antigenic properties of which differ according to the stage (germinative or maturating) and to the type (orthokeratosis, parakeratosis, mucosa, etc.) of differentiation.

We have previously found that patients undergoing a bone marrow graft for aplastic anemia or leukemia had, in their serum, antibodies (IgG) reacting with epidermal cells (1). As shown by indirect immunofluorescence and immunoperoxidase staining these antibodies were found to be directed against the cytoplasm of the epidermal cells (i.e. keratinocytes) (2,3). In this report we confirm the frequency of 'keratino-cyte cytoplasmic antibodies' (KCA) after bone marrow trans-plantation and demonstrate that KCA react with cytoplasmic components closely related to the stage and to the type of keratinocyte differentiation.

MATERIAL AND METHODS

Sera

Sera were obtained (1) from 45 patients undergoing a bone marrow graft for aplastic anemia (36 cases) or leukemia (9 cases). Serum samples were obtained each week and processed for skin antibody content (see below). A total of 383 sera were studied; (2) from 920 subjects with various skin dis-eases attending the dermatologic clinic. A total of 951 sera were studied; (3) from 45 healthy donors (the donors of the bone marrow grafts); and (4) from 31 patients with idio-

[*]This work was supported by grants from ATP INSERM 78 99 and E.R.A. CNRS 625.

TABLE 1. Significant titers of keratinocyte cytoplasmic antibodies (KCA) detected by indirect immunofluorescence on malpighian substrates are more frequent after a bone marrow graft than in the other conditions studied

		Patients with KCA (≥ 1/10)			Sera with KCA* (≥ 1/10)		
		Number	of..	%	Number	of..	%
I	Normal controls	0	20	0	–	–	–
	Patients with skin diseases	27	920	3	30	951	3
	Healthy bone marrow donors from:						
II	families of aplastic anemias	5	36	14	–	–	–
	families of leukemias	0	9	–	–	–	–
	Patients with aplastic anemia	3	31	11			
	of which: ... treated with ATG	2	13	15	16	153	10.5
III	After a bone marrow graft (AA: 36, Leuk.: 9)	29	45	65	92	383	24

χ^2: (I ≠ II; P < 0.01); (II ≠ III; P < 0.001); *follow-up studies.

pathic aplastic anemia treated with androgens (18 cases) or antithymocyte globulins (13 cases) (Table 1).

Techniques

Standard technique The sera were routinely studied by indirect immunofluorescence (IIF) as previously described (1). Three substrates were used: blood group O human skin specimens, rabbit lip (see below) and rabbit esophagus sections. The specificity of the staining has been previously demonstrated (1,4). The indirect immunoperoxidase technique has been found to give similar results (3).

Study of the relationship with keratinocyte differentiation Previous results (4) have suggested that the type of differentiation of the substrate used for IIF was an important factor. Therefore we studied the pattern of reaction of 10 sera containing KCA obtained from 8 patients after a bone marrow graft on several substrates with a well-defined type of differentiation: human skin and rabbit skin specimens for orthokeratinization, vaginal sections from castrated rats treated with estradiol for parakeratinization, and human and rabbit esophagus sections for mucosa. Moreover, we used specimens in which several types of keratinocyte differentiation were occurring on a single section. (1) Rabbit lip sections, obtained from the junctional zone between skin and mucosa. Such a section gave, on a single specimen, areas of mucosa, parakeratotic and orthokeratotic epithelium with well-defined junctional zones between the 3 types of keratinocyte differentiation. (2) Mouse tail epidermis, which gave on a single specimen areas of parakeratotic and of orthokeratotic epithelium. The transitional zones between the 2 epidermal structures were unusually sharp. (3) Vertical and horizontal serial sections of human scalp, in which the staining pattern obtained by IIF could be studied in regard to the external root sheath of hairs below and above the orifice of the sebaceous gland duct.

The organ specificity of KCA was studied on the following substrates: liver, kidney, spleen, thyroid, gallbladder, pylorus stomach (man, rabbit), colon duodenum, brain, adrenal glands, and thymus (rabbit).

RESULTS

Frequency of KCA

KCA (IgG) were found to occur significantly more often in patients undergoing a bone marrow graft. Sequential studies have demonstrated that the occurrence of KCA was not strictly correlated with a GVHR. Patients with aplastic anemia, before any graft, and healthy bone marrow donors (from the family of the grafted patients) were found to produce KCA more frequently than normal controls or patients with various skin diseases.

Organ specificity

Sera with KCA were not found to react by IIF with the cytoplasm of cells present in other tissues. Two sera (Nos. 2
and 5, Tables 2 and 3) reacted with Hassaal corpuscles of
thymus sections; this part of the organ is known to undergo
keratinization.

Staining patterns

Relationships with keratinocyte differentiation:

Relationships with the stage of keratinocyte differentiation Two staining patterns were observed: staining of the
cytoplasm of basal cells (Fig. 1) and a staining of cells
of the prickle, granular and horny layers, i.e. the upper
layers (Fig. 2). The former represents the germinative
(or proliferative) compartment in stratified squamous
epithelia, the latter corresponds to the differentiating
(or maturating) compartment.

Relationships with the type of keratinocyte differentiation
Some sera were found to react only with the cells belonging
either to an orthokeratinized, a parakeratinized or to a
mucous epithelium (Tables 2 and 3). This was observed in
the proliferative as well as in the maturating compartment.
Most characteristically there were abrupt interruptions of
the staining (basal or upper) in the sections showing distinct types of differentiation on a single specimen; the
abrupt changes were strictly located at the junctional
zones between either ortho- and parakeratinization or between parakeratinization and mucosa (Fig. 3). The changes
have been reproduced repeatedly. The external root sheath
of hairs was found to express antigenic properties similar
to those of orthokeratinized epithelia above the orifice
of the sebaceous gland but to have distinct antigens below
this orifice (details in Ref. 5).

DISCUSSION

In a larger series (1) we confirmed that patients undergoing
a bone marrow transplantation frequently produce IgG antibodies against the cytoplasm of epidermal cells. This fact
probably reflects the consequence of skin injury after a
bone marrow graft whatever its cause may be (for example,
GVHR; drugs) (1). The skin injury would liberate epidermal
(hidden?) antigens. Problems in T and B lymphocyte cooperation in these patients would also play a role.
    KCA do not seem to be involved in the induction of any
skin lesion after bone marrow grafting: they are never
found in vivo (1), and they do not penetrate into living
keratinocytes (in preparation). At present we cannot obtain
any evidence for a strong correlation between KCA and GVHR
(6). However, KCA were found to detect an antigenic poly-
morphism in human epidermis (7) which was not related to

216

TABLE 2. Results of indirect immunofluorescence, with 10 sera obtained from 8 patients after a bone marrow transplantation, on several stratified squamous epithelia involved in distinct types of differentiation

Types of differentiation	Germinative compartments (basal staining)														
	Orthokeratotic			Parakeratotic			Mucosa			ERS (I)			ERS (II)		
Origin of the substrate	HSK	RL	MT	RL	MT	RV	HO	RL	RO	HSK	HSc	RL	HSK	HSc	RL
Number of experiments	50	20	7	20	7	6	3	20	50	50	5	20	50	5	20
Sera Nos. Titers															
1 .200	−	−	−	−	−	−	o	−	−	−	−	−	+	+	+
2 .100	−	−	−	−	−	−	+	+	+	−	−	−	+	+	+
3 .100	−	−	−	−	−	−	o	+	+	−	−	−	+	+	+
4 .100	−	−	−	−	−	−	o	+	+	−	−	−	−	−	−
5 .50	−	−	−	−	−	o	o	+	+	−	−	−	−	−	−
6 .100	−	−	−	+	+	(−)	o	+	+	−	−	−	+	+	+
7 .100	−	−	−	+	+	o	o	+	+	−	−	−	+	+	+
8 .200	+	+	+	+	+	+	o	+	+	+	+	+	+	+	+
9 .200	+	+	+	+	+	+	o	+	+	+	+	+	+	+	+
10 .50	+	+	+	+	+	+	+	+	+	+	+	+	+	+	+

Only the reaction with the germinative compartments of each substrate (resulting in a basal staining, see Fig. 1) is quoted. HSK: human skin; RL: Rabbit lip; MT: mouse tail; RV: rat vagina; HO: human oesophagus; RO: rabbit oesophagus; HSc: human scalp; ERS: external root sheath of hairs, (I): above the sebaceous duct orifice and (II): under this orifice. (+) basal staining. (−) no basal staining. (o) not done.

It can be seen that when a serum was found to react with the germinative compartment of one type of differentiation it reacted with substrates of distinct origin but involved in a similar differentiation; when a serum did not react with a substrate involved in one type of differentiation it did not react with the substrates involved in the same type of differentiation. Therefore, the antigenic specificities expressed in the cytoplasm of the keratinocytes in the terminative compartments differ whether the cell program is directed toward either ortho-keratinization, parakeratinization, mucosa or external root sheath of hairs.

TABLE 3. Results of indirect immunofluorescence, with 10 sera obtained from 8 patients after a bone marrow transplantation, on several stratified squamous epithelia involved in distinct types of differentiation

	Maturating compartments (upper staining)														
Type of differentiation	Orthokeratotic			Parakeratotic			Mucosa			ERS (I)			ERS (II)		
Origin of the substrate	HSK	RL	MT	RL	MT	RV	HO	RL	RO	HSK	HSc	RL	HSK	HSc	RL
Number of experiments	50	20	7	20	7	6	3	20	50	50	5	20	50	5	20
Sera Nos. Titers															
1 . 200	–	–	–	–	–	–	o	–	–	–	–	–	–	–	–
2 . 100	+	+	+	+	+	+	–	–	–	+	+	+	–	–	–
3 . 100	+	+	+	–	–	–	o	–	–	+	+	+	–	–	–
4 . 100	+	+	+	–	–	–	o	–	–	+	+	+	o	o	o
5 . 50	+	+	+	–	–	o	o	–	–	+	+	+	o	o	o
6 . 100	–	–	+	+	+	(–)	o	+	+	–	–	–	–	–	–
7 . 100	–	–	+	+	+	o	o	+	+	–	–	–	–	–	–
8 . 200	–	–	–	–	–	(+)	o	–	–	–	–	–	+	+	+
9 . 200	–	–	–	–	–	o	o	–	–	–	–	–	+	+	+
10 . 50	–	–	–	–	–	o	–	–	–	–	–	–	–	–	–

For abbreviations, see Table 2.
Only the reaction with the maturating compartments (resulting in an upper staining, see Fig. 2) is quoted. When a serum was found to react with the maturating compartment of one type of differentiation it reacted with the substrates of distinct origins but involved in a similar type of differentiation and vice versa. Therefore, the antigenic specificities expressed in the cytoplasm of the keratinocytes in the maturating compartments differ whether the cell is involved either in an orthokeratinized, parakeratinized, mucosal, or external root sheath type of differentiation.

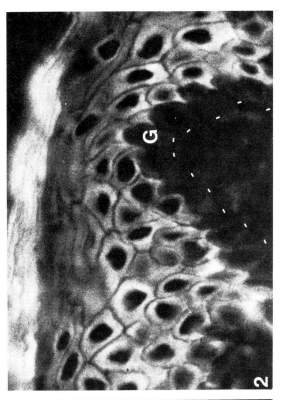

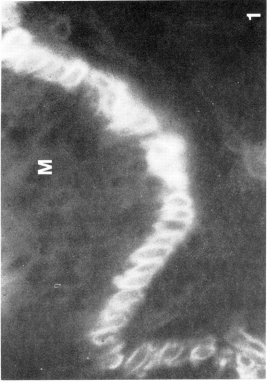

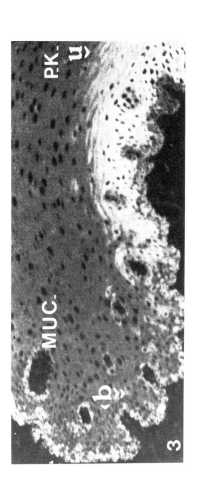

the blood groups or HL-A antigens (2). Further work is needed in order to study the immunogenetic aspects of these findings. KCA may occur in normal subjects but in very low titers (8). We have found that, in healthy subjects from families of patients with aplastic anemia (bone marrow donors), the occurrence of KCA in significant titers (1/10-1/50) was high. This has not been explained and has to be confirmed in a larger series.

The most important finding was that KCA were found to react with cytoplasmic components linked to the stage and the type of keratinocyte maturation.

Keratinocytes are the main cellular components of stratified squamous epithelia (SSE). In SSE 2 stages and several types of differentiation can be distinguished. The keratinocyte in the unicellular basal cell layer, while it cannot be considered structurally or functionally undifferentiated, is the least differentiated cell of the tissue. Mitosis occurs only in this basal layer, which is called the germinative or proliferative compartment of SSE. The cell layers situated above the germinative compartment are made of non-dividing cells involved only in a progressive process of maturation. Several types of maturation are known for keratinocytes: full keratinization (orthokeratinization), partial keratinization (parakeratinization), non-keratinization (mucosa), etc.

We have demonstrated that the KCA react either with

Fig. 1. Indirect immunofluorescence with serum No. 8 (see Table 2) on rabbit lip section, mucosal side. Staining of the cytoplasm of the basal cell layer (germinative compartment). No staining in the upper cell layers (maturating compartment, M). The cytoplasm of basal cells is not abundant and the areas stained are smaller than in the upper compartments (see Fig. 2). However, the cytoplasmic localization of the staining has been established by means of immunoperoxidase techniques which allow a higher magnification (3).

Fig. 2. Indirect immunofluorescence with serum No. 2 (see Table 3) on human skin section (orthokeratosis). Staining of the upper cell layer (maturating compartment). No staining of the basal cell layer (germinative compartment, G). The basal pole unstained basal cells has been underlined.

Fig. 3. Indirect immunofluorescence with serum No. 2 (see Tables 2 and 3) on rabbit lip specimen. The section has been made in order to give a single specimen area of orthokeratosis, parakeratosis and mucosa. The figure represents the junctional area between mucosa (MUC) and parakeratosis (PK). It can be seen that there is a basal staining (b) on the mucosal side and a progressive upper staining (u) on the parakeratotic side. The change in the staining distribution corresponds to the change in the type of differentiation. (Serum No. 2 has been found to contain antibodies to the germinative compartment of mucosa and to the maturating compartment of parakeratosis, see Tables 2 and 3.)

germinative or maturating cells. Moreover, KCA react either with cells programmed for, or involved in, orthokeratinization, parakeratinization, mucosal differentiation, etc. Therefore, keratinocytes express distinct cytoplasmic specificities according to the stage and the type of maturation. The concept that SSE are made of subunits of cells expressing distinct antigenic properties has not been considered previously. It may prove to be useful to study the antigenic composition of SSE with regard to skin and bone marrow grafts.

REFERENCES

1. Saurat, J.H., Bonnetblanc, J.M., Gluckman, E., Didierjean, L. and Puissant, A. (1976): Skin antibodies in bone marrow transplanted patients. Clin. exp. Derm., 1, 377-384.
2. Saurat, J.H., Gluckman, E., Didierjean, L., Andersen, E., Sockeel, F. and Puissant, A. (1977): Cytoplasmic and HL-A antigens in human epidermis. Brit. J. Derm., 96, 603-608.
3. Janin Mercier, A., Saurat, J.H. and Didierjean, L. (1979): Epidermal cytoplasmic antibodies are also detected by indirect immunoperoxydase staining. Arch. derm. Res., in press.
4. Saurat, J.H., Didierjean, L., Beucher, F. and Gluckman, E. (1978): Immunofluorescent tracing of cytoplasmic components involved in keratinocyte differentiation. Brit. J. Derm., 98, 155-163.
5. Saurat, J.H., Didierjean, L. and Gluckman, E. (1978): Antigènes de différenciation du kératinocyte. II Spécificités exprimées dans le compartiment basal de la gaine épithéliale externe du poil et non exprimées dans l'épiderme. C. R. Acad. Sci. (Paris), 286, 1273-1276.
6. Saurat, J.H. and Gluckman, E. (1977): The lichen planus like eruption after bone marrow transplantation. A manifestation of the graft versus host disease. Clin. exp. Derm., 2, 335-344.
7. Saurat, J.H., Didierjean, L., Gluckman, E., Lauraine Pujade, M.D. and Puissant, A. (1977): Studies on epidermal cytoplasmic antibodies. J. invest. Derm., 68, 245.
8. Bystryn, J.C., Abel, E. and Weidman, A. (1973): Antibodies against the cytoplasm of human epidermal cells. Arch. Derm., 108, 241-245.

AUTHOR INDEX